Homeopathy

Homeopathy

How It *Really* Works

Jay W. Shelton

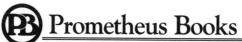 Prometheus Books
59 John Glenn Drive
Amherst, New York 14228-2197

Published 2004 by Prometheus Books

Inquiries should be addressed to
Prometheus Books
59 John Glenn Drive
Amherst, New York 14228–2197
VOICE: 716–691–0133, ext. 207
FAX: 716–564–2711
WWW.PROMETHEUSBOOKS.COM

08 07 06 05 04   5 4 3 2 1

Library of Congress Cataloging-in-Publication Data

Shelton, Jay, 1942–
    Homeopathy : how it really works / by Jay W. Shelton.
        p. ; cm.
    Includes bibliographical references.
    ISBN 1–59102–109–X (pbk. : alk. paper)
    1. Homeopathy.
    [DNLM: 1. Homeopathy—methods. 2. Holistic Health. 3. Materia Medica—therapeutic use. WB 930 S545h 2003] I. Title.

RX71.S485 2003
615.5'32—dc21

                                                                    2003010925

Printed in the United States on acid-free paper

Contents

Acknowledgments

I am grateful to the following people for useful feedback on all or parts of the manuscript: Iris Bell, Ph.D., M.D.; Anthony Campbell, M.D.; Julian Winston; David Riley, M.D.; Nancy Nylander; John Shelton, Ph.D.; Heidi Lynch; Don Feinberg, M.D.; Sharon Angert; Reed Jackson; Jeremy Bradford; Anita Herron; David Kern; Ryan Leary; and Ann Dasburg. I am especially indebted to Jim Klemmer, whose patient perseverance in trying to help me understand the homeopathic perspective enabled us to have stimulating and productive dialogue despite differing perspectives. I acknowledge the help of all these people, and none bears responsibility for any errors in this book. And, finally, I thank my wife, Katherine, for making the whole project possible.

Introduction

Homeopathy is an approach to health care based primarily on the concept that a patient can be cured by properly prepared minute doses of a substance which, when given to healthy people, induces the patient's symptoms. This book is a study of homeopathy, not a self-help guide for using homeopathy. It is primarily an application of critical thinking and the methods of science to homeopathy.

Homeopathy was developed about two hundred years ago by a German physician, Samuel Hahnemann (1755–1843), at a time when there was great dissatisfaction with conventional health care. Medical practice was not very effective, and many treatments, such as blood-letting, were detrimental to health. After about a century of strong growth, homeopathy entered a deep decline in the United States that was roughly coincident with the rise of science and the understanding of the biological causes of many common diseases and ailments.

Over the last few decades, the popularity of homeopathy has increased dramatically, both in the United States and worldwide. Annual U.S. sales of remedies increased by 500 percent between 1987 and 1999, and worldwide sales in 1999 were about $1.5 billion.[1]

Homeopathic care can be provided by professional **homeopaths**, or patients can self-prescribe. The self-prescriber market, for remedies one can buy at grocery and drug stores without a prescription, is much larger than the prescription market. Most of the remedies are in the form of tiny, round sugar pills with names that reveal the condition to be treated: "Sinus," "Alertness," or "Constipation." Another class of homeopathic remedies has names like "Sabina 30C," "Hep. sulph. calc. 30C," and "Arnica montana 6X." To know which remedy is needed for which condition requires some homework, and dozens of books are designed to help the caregiver understand homeopathy and select the right remedy.

Homeopathy is hard to define. There is substantial dissension within homeopathy over what "authentic" homeopathy is and over which practices have been "verified." This book deals primarily with what has come to be called **classical homeopathy** but includes examples and discussion of what some would call the creative and forward-looking part of the field, and others would call the wandering and perhaps lost fringe.

Some homeopaths are overtly proud of how unscientific homeopathy is; they see it as an art, an intuitive healing system which they believe science will never explain. Classical homeopaths, however, see the field as solidly grounded in science. They chide the New Agers for not following "proven scientific methods." And therein lies a major disconnect; a close look reveals substantial discrepancies between classical homeopaths' and scientists' view of what science is.

How can there be such a wide range of views within homeopathy on its scientific aspects? Some self-declared homeopaths have essentially no formal education in science, while a few are M.D.s or Ph.D.s. Some have formal education in homeopathy and some have none. There are no generally accepted training, degree, or certification requirements for homeopaths. Thus the term "homeopath" as commonly used is ill-defined.

Today's resurgence in interest is again caused in part by dissatisfaction with conventional medical care. Many treatments are seen as invasive and uncomfortable, and the whole system can be impersonal. The shift toward homeopathy is coincident with growing public mistrust of and distaste for conventional medicine as well as for science generally. Homeopathy is perceived as natural, effective, safe, and free of side effects, and its delivery by professional homeopaths is viewed as gentle, caring, and patient. What more could one ask? We want it to be true.

But *is* it true? Homeopathy is still looking for a plausible mechanism that explains how homeopathic remedies should work, particularly the many very dilute remedies with none of the **original medicinal molecules** remaining. But this shortcoming is not fatal, as science need not know *how* remedies work in order to use its tools, clinical trials, to determine *whether* the remedies work. The data from such trials are mixed; some studies support homeopathic remedies and some do not. The studies with the highest methodological quality appear to be least supportive.

Although most patients who visit homeopaths are better as a consequence, the remedies are not necessarily the cause. The role of the **placebo response**, for example, is often underappreciated. Homeopaths tell their patients that unhealthy lifestyles can block the remedy from working; patients are urged to improve their diets, get more exercise and rest, and reduce stress in their lives. Homeopaths sometimes urge simultaneous non-homeopathic treatments, as well as the cessation of treatments with uncomfortable or harmful side effects. The caring and optimistic attitude of the professional homeopath can have a significant effect on the patient's psychological health. Homeopathic patients will often improve due to these proven mechanisms, but homeopaths almost always give all the credit to their remedies.

Homeopathic theory is weak from a scientific point of view, in part because it has many vaguely or circularly defined concepts. It has multiple explanations for some of the same patient outcomes and has exceptions to many of its "laws." Homeopaths claim that their patients may get better or worse, sooner or later, with old or new symptoms, and that the bad as well as the good is caused by the remedies. This claim may well be nonfalsifiable and hence not scientifically testable. Another scientific weakness is homeopathy's reliance on its founder and his written word to settle disputes and factual questions; Hahnemann and his writings are held in almost religious reverence by most homeopaths.

If homeopathic remedies are not the active part of homeopathic health benefits, then the most interesting question is how so many intelligent homeopaths and patients could have misinterpreted their observations for so long. Understanding the difference between people's individual internal reality and the external reality of nature is key. This book explores the external reality of homeopaths' internal realities.

NOTE

1. J. P. Borneman, "Homeopathy, Progress and Promise: A Critical Perspective," Blackie Memorial Lecture, 2001, *British Homeopathic Journal* 90, no. 4 (2001): 204–13. Some homeopaths believe that $1.5 billion is an overestimate.

1. *Introduction to Classical Homeopathy*

This chapter is devoted to the foundations of classical homeopathy, primarily for the benefit of readers who have little prior knowledge of the subject. It provides background for the more analytical approach found in the rest of the book. A critical look at one topic—the **vital force**—is also included.

TWO CASES

Two cases illustrate how easy it is for a critical thinker to become interested in homeopathy. The first case is described by the patient's mother:

Acute First-Degree Burns . . .

We were visiting friends for a barbecue with our four-year-old son, Kailin. . . . Kailin got too close to it [the grill] and touched the bottom of the kettle with his elbow. . . . I ran to him as he screamed in pain and saw a large patch of skin already changing color. Luckily, I knew these friends had just that week purchased a homeopathic home kit. I told them to get it quickly as I held my ice-filled glass on his arm, which helped the pain a little. Within a couple of minutes the kit arrived and I chose the remedy Cantharis [prepared from Spanish fly] and gave Kailin a dose. Within two or three minutes the pain stopped and we all watched over the next fifteen minutes as the skin started to lighten in color. I repeated the remedy several times, whenever he said the pain was starting to return. By the next day the burn was all but gone and totally cleared in two days. We were all amazed that no blisters ever formed.[1]

Several questions come to mind. If the burn had not been treated homeopathically, would its progress have been any different? Why were they amazed that no blisters formed given that the author describes the injury as a first-degree burn, which, by definition, does not involve blisters? Could any of the reduction in pain be explained by the icing, the distraction of a sweet pill, and the attention of expectant adults, or by the unassisted natural evolution of pain and healing? Why are patients and homeopaths so easily convinced that the remedy was the cause of the pain reduction and cure?

The second case, the treatment of cancer, is described by a professional homeopath:

Female, 39 years, presented with a 1 cm lump in the right breast, lower quadrant, that had been diagnosed as cancerous. . . . The patient was overweight [and] could eat only a little at a time, but liked pastries; she was easily chilled but craved fresh air. She was gentle by nature; easily felt hurt or slighted; and was low-spirited, mornings and evenings—all symptoms pointing to Pulsatilla. Prescription: Week 1: Pulsatilla 200C— daily, Plussing Method.[2]

It is interesting that a serious disease like cancer is being treated homeopathically. It is also curious that the woman's likes, dislikes, and personality are used in selecting the first prescription. The remedy Pulsatilla is derived from a flowering plant, and its 200C form is diluted by a factor of 10^{400} (1 followed by 400 zeros). None of the original plant molecules remain in this remedy after so much dilution. Yet homeopaths report remarkable cures and believe that their most dilute remedies are the most potent. The **plussing** method mentioned in the passage involves additional dilution and stirring or shaking of a liquid remedy before each dose, which is thought by homeopaths to further increase the remedy's potency.

These two cases illustrate just a few of the many interesting aspects of homeopathy:

- A tendency of homeopaths to ignore all other possible causes of improved health other than their remedies
- Use of a patient's normal personality to select a remedy to treat her cancer
- Use of remedies so dilute that none of the original substance is left
- Belief that even with no molecules left, further dilution accompanied by stirring or shaking makes the remedy even stronger.

Clearly homeopathy is different and is intriguing!

DR. HAHNEMANN AND THE LAW OF SIMILARS

A few centuries ago, many medical treatments in the Western world had no curative value and were even harmful. Practices such as bloodletting, induced sweating, diarrhea, vomiting, or dehydration, and administering nearly toxic doses of poisons such as mercury and arsenic were common.

In the late 1700s, a German physician named Samuel Hahnemann sought to develop a system of medicine that was gentler and more effective than contemporary medical practice. He knew that mercury was commonly used to treat syphilis and noted a similarity between syphilis symptoms and those of mercury poisoning. He wondered whether there were other similar cases of diseases that were cured by substances that themselves produced the disease symptoms in healthy people. Hahnemann knew that bark from the Peruvian cinchona tree was used to treat malaria; the bark contains quinine, which is still used today to treat malaria. However, there were no data on the symptoms of cinchona poisoning. Consequently, Hahnemann decided to investigate these symptoms by consuming the bark extract. He reported symptoms that were very similar to those of malaria patients, including numbness, thirst, coldness, tiredness, and aches. After a while, Hahnemann's symptoms cleared. He repeated this experiment on himself twice more and reported the same results.

Hahnemann wondered if he had found a universal principle: a substance that causes particular symptoms in a healthy person cures a sick person with the same symptoms. After apparently confirming this relation for some other medications in use at the time, Hahnemann expanded his investigations to include materials never used before as medicines and reported the same pattern; substances seemed to induce in healthy people the same symptoms that they seemed to cure in sick people. This is Hahne-

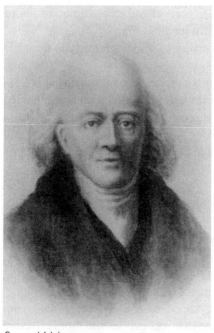

Samuel Hahnemann.
Photo courtesy of Julian Winston.

mann's **Law of Similars**, the core of homeopathy.

This similarity principle was not new. The Greeks, the Romans (Galen), and Paracelsus in the Renaissance had formulated similar concepts, but Hahnemann was probably the first to conduct systematic investigations of the effects of potential remedies on healthy people.

THE SINGLE REMEDY: THE SIMILLIMUM

It was common in Hahnemann's time for physicians to prescribe multiple simultaneous treatments. Hahnemann believed that every health problem could be cured by a single remedy: "In no case of cure is it necessary to employ more than a *single simple* medicinal substance at one time with a patient. *For this reason alone, it is inadmissible to do so*."[3] He felt that the single homeopathic remedy that best matched the patient's symptoms, what he called the **simillimum**, was the most effective treatment. Over time, other remedies might be called for in response to the changing symptoms of the patient, but only one remedy should be given at a time.

The Importance of Succussion

Concerned about the strong side effects of Cinchona and other remedies, many of which were toxic, Hahnemann was inclined to use the smallest dose (**minimum dose**) that was effective. After trying more dilute forms of the same remedies, he reported that the side effects decreased, but so did the curative powers unless the solution was also *succussed* by a specific type of agitation.

A story is often told about the origins of **succussion**. Supposedly, Hahnemann noted that remedies carried in his horse-drawn carriage or his saddle bags to a patient's home seemed to be more effective than remedies given to patients at his office. He hypothesized that the jiggling of the remedies during his travels made the medicines stronger. Henceforth, when diluting remedies, Hahnemann did not just stir or swirl them but shook them by pounding the remedy bottle repeatedly against a leather-bound book.[4] He called this process *succussion* (in translation from the German *Schütteln*) and believed that it made the remedies more potent.

Hahnemann concluded that side effects could be eliminated with sufficient dilution, and that the **potency** of the remedy actually increased with additional dilution, as long as the remedies were succussed at each dilution. Neither dilution alone nor vigorous shaking alone made remedies more potent. The combined processes of dilution and succession is called **potentization.** In this way, Hahnemann felt he had achieved his objective of creating remedies with strong healing powers and essentially no side effects.

WHAT KINDS OF AILMENTS CAN HOMEOPATHY TREAT?

The public knows homeopathy best for its ability to assist recovery from **acute ailments**, defined as health problems that are always quick and often severe; they arise quickly but do not last long. Acute ailments include stings, blisters, bruises, cold sores, coughs, diarrhea, fever, indigestion, cuts, sunburn, colds, flu, sore throats, and occasional headaches. These ailments are self-limiting in that the patient generally recovers from them without intervention, or the patient dies.

In contrast to acute ailments, **chronic conditions** develop more slowly and last longer. Examples that homeopaths claim to be able to treat include arthritis, obesity, diabetes, hypertension, migraine headaches, eating disorders, torn ligaments, Alzheimer's disease, multiple sclerosis, epilepsy, sciatica, Parkinson's disease, and asthma.

Practitioners consider treatment of chronic conditions most successful if the condition disappears and never returns, but lessening of symptom intensity, better tolerance of symptoms, and even a better outlook on life with no change in physical symptoms are also considered positive outcomes.

Homeopaths also treat psychological conditions such as phobias, eating disorders, depression, attention deficit disorder, jealousy, the psychological effects of childhood sexual abuse, compulsive hand washing, and even the "deep-seated belief that one deserves divine wrath."[5] Some homeopaths also claim to be able to treat cancer, alcoholism, and criminal behavior.

Most homeopaths suggest using conventional medicine for such conditions as broken bones, AIDS, hepatitis, and severe burns, while concurrently using homeopathy to hasten recovery and reduce pain from such afflictions.

TREATING THE INDIVIDUAL, NOT JUST THE DISEASE

Homeopaths treat the **whole person**, not just the nominal disease or ailment. If the patient's main complaint is painful fingers, whether or not the patient worries about what others think of him may be important in the remedy selection process. If one is seeking relief from depression, it may matter whether one loves or hates fish. *All* of the patient's symptoms are relevant as the homeopath selects the remedy, and the term **symptom** is interpreted very broadly. Because the remedies are **individualized** to each patient, in homeopathy there is no "remedy x" that is always used for "condition y." In addition, *all* illness symptoms, not just the main complaint that caused the patient to seek help, are supposed to go away after homeopathic treatment.[6]

In a sense, homeopathy does not recognize the bacterial and viral causes of disease. The real cause, according to homeopathy, is some deeper susceptibility of the patient. Medications such as penicillin that rid the body of certain bacteria do not address that deeper level; the correct homeopathic remedy is thought to strengthen the body's resistance to the bacteria so that the disease will not recur. Thus homeopaths claim to achieve "real" **cures** and characterize conventional medicine as often just "suppressing" symptoms—reducing fever, making a muscle less sore, drying up a runny nose.

REMEDY SOURCES

Homeopaths sometimes classify remedies according to their origins (see table 1.1).

Table 1.1. Primary Source Types for Homeopathic Remedies

Classification	Comment	Examples
Minerals and Elements		Gold, salt, calcium carbonate
Plants		Coffee, deadly nightshade, belladonna, onion
Animals		Cuttlefish, honeybee, wolf milk
Nosodes	Remedies prepared from diseased tissue; causative agents such as bacteria, viruses, yeast, parasites; or excretions and secretions. Sterilization is part of the process.	Cancer tumor, pus, saliva from rabid animal
Imponderables	Remedies whose starting material is not atoms or molecules.	X rays, light, magnetic field

Remedies based on plants or animals may be made from the entire plant or animal, or just a part. For instance, Apis mellifica starts with ground up whole honeybees, whereas Apis venenum purum is made from just the venom of a bee.

The list of source types in table 1.1 is not exhaustive. Some additional remedy types are described in *The Homeopathic Pharmacopoeia of the United States* (**HPUS**),[7] the official authority on homeopathic remedies in the United States.

The total number of remedies in use throughout the world is probably around ten thousand. In the future, there may be many more remedies; homeopaths believe that *everything* is a potential remedy. The number of remedies officially recognized by the HPUS is between one thousand and two thousand. The number of remedies in common use is smaller— probably hundreds.

NOT ALL REMEDIES COME FROM HERBS AND FLOWERS

Some people think of homeopathic remedies as being made from entirely natural, pleasant, and safe materials such as edible herbs, flowers, berries, and roots. The connotation is pastoral and peaceful, but not all remedies fit this image.

Some remedies are made from unpleasant substances. If one can imagine it, there may well be a remedy made from it, including such things as feces, pus, vomit, cancer tumors, warts, dental plaque, putrid meat, rotten potatoes, and insects. A nineteenth-century homeopath described collecting raw material for the remedy Psorinum this way: "In the Autumn of 1880 I collected pus from the itch pustule of a young and otherwise healthy Negro, who had been infected [with scabies] . . . The pustules were full, large and yellow. . . . I opened all the mature unscratched pustules for several days in succession and collected the pus in a vial with alcohol."[8]

Herbs are natural but not always safe. Homeopathic remedies are made from such noxious plants as poison ivy, belladonna, hemlock, and hashish. Remedies are also made from some potent animal poisons, such as venom from snakes. Others are made from strong chemicals such as insecticides, solvents, and disinfectants; toxic elements such as arsenic, lead, and mercury; and radioactive materials such as uranium, radium, and plutonium. Thus the safety of some homeopathic remedies is due not to their starting materials but to the dilutions, to which sterilization is added in the case of materials containing pathogenic microbes.

Many remedies are not pain-free for the donor animals. For instance, the scorpion remedy starts with an injection into the rectum of a live scorpion.[9] The making of Cimex lectularius starts with crushing live bedbugs. Serum anguilae requires surgical entry into a live eel. Scolopendra centipede starts by making a tincture from live centipedes.

Some remedies require much exertion on the part of living creatures. Tela aranearum is made from the web of garden spiders: "The insect [sic] is made to run along a hoop and then made to fall by shaking, so that it hangs by its own thread. The hoop is then rotated and as much thread as possible extracted. . . . [I]n order to extract one grain several hours of strenuous work (involving many spiders) are necessary."[10]

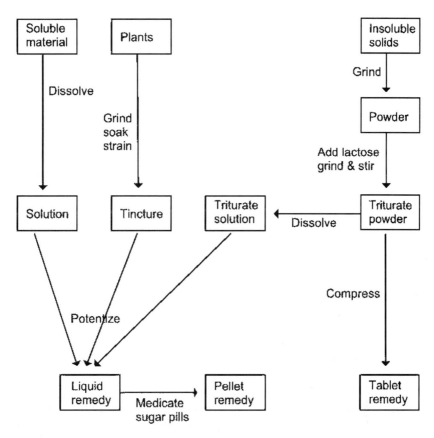

Figure 1.1. Outline of remedy-manufacturing processes.

REMEDY PREPARATION

The overall process of making homeopathic remedies is outlined in figure 1.1. The most unusual aspect is repeated dilution of the starting material and the shaking succussion of each dilution ("potentize" in figure 1.1). The process is somewhat complex and tightly prescribed by the HPUS. The following examples illustrate key features. (For more details, see appendix 1).

The starting material for a Belladonna remedy is the entire belladonna plant just as it is beginning to flower. The plant is ground up and placed in a sealed jar with alcohol and water. This process is like making tea except for the lack of heat; some of the molecules in the plant dissolve into the liquid. The alcohol helps both as a solvent and as a preservative. The process typically requires a few weeks, during which the jar is occasionally shaken. The liquid tea is then filtered from the solid plant material, yielding what is called the **tincture** or **mother tincture**. This is also a 1X liquid remedy since it is in some sense (see appendix 1) ten times more dilute than the original plant ("**X**" being the Roman numeral for ten).[11]

Usually the tincture is further processed before use. If the tincture is diluted by a factor of 10 (by combining one part of the tincture with 9 parts water or alcohol) and the result is succussed (figure 1.2), the result is called a 2X liquid **attenuation** and is also essentially the same as a 2X liquid remedy. (*Attenuation* is the name for the result of each dilution-plus-succussion stage.)[12] If the 2X attenuation is diluted by a factor of 10 and then succussed, it becomes a 3X attenuation or remedy. The process is often carried on up to 30X. There are ten times fewer belladonna molecules at each stage. A 12X remedy has been diluted twelve times by a factor of ten and is thus 10^{12} or 1,000,000,000,000 times more dilute than the original material. X remedies are also called **decimal remedies**.

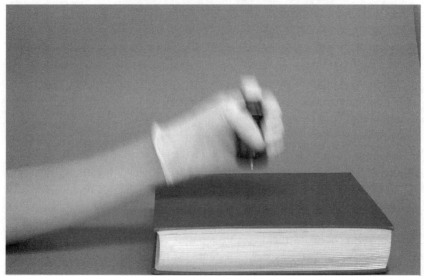

Figure 1.2. The succussion process.

The tincture can also be diluted by a factor of one hundred instead of ten at each stage, and such remedies are given designation such as 1C, 2C, 3C since *C* is the Roman numeral for 100.[13] These **C** or **centesimal remedies** are made all the way up to 100,000C and occasionally beyond. At some point, not one of the original molecules is left, as will be discussed in chapter 3. (Homeopaths usually use a shorthand notation for centesimal remedies of 1,000C and higher. 1M is an alternative designation for 1,000C, 10M for 10,000C, etc. **M** is the Roman numeral for 1000.)

Some homeopathic medicinal materials are not soluble in water or alcohol, including substances such as granite, diamond, and platinum. Making remedies from these materials starts with grinding and solid-phase dilution in a process called **trituration** (figure 1.3). One part (by mass) of the ground raw material is mixed with ninety-nine parts lactose, and the mixture is vigorously ground and stirred in a mortar with a pestle. One part of this ground mixture is then mixed with ninety-nine parts more lactose, and the process is repeated. One final repetition of this process results in a finely ground material that is one million times more dilute than the original material. At this stage, it is considered a 3C attenuation; its dilution is the same as the 3C remedies discussed earlier. This material is then treated as though it were soluble,[14] in that it is "dissolved" in water so that further liquid attenuations can be made from it. Alternatively, further attenuations may be obtained by continued successive triturations. At any stage of trituration, the material can be compressed into remedy pills.

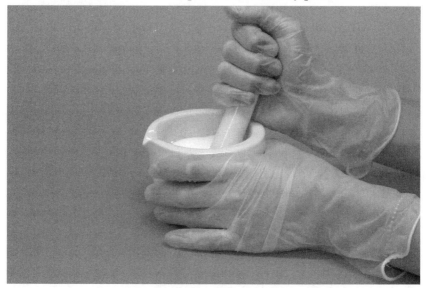

Figure 1.3. The process of trituration.

Homeopaths use two other terms, potentization and **dynamization**, for these liquid or solid attenuation processes; these terms convey homeopaths' belief that the process of dilution and succession (or trituration) brings out the healing *power* of the original materials.

The final homeopathic remedies can be prepared in a variety of forms (figure 1.4). Ingestible forms may be based on a water and alcohol mixture (usually 20 percent alcohol to assure that no microbes can survive or grow), glycerin, powders (lactose or sucrose), sugar pills or tablets, or rice paper wafers. Topical preparations may be ointments, lotions, gels, or cerates. More specialized forms include ophthalmic solutions, nasal solutions, suppositories, lozenges, and ampoules of injectable remedies. For the common sugar-pill form of homeopathic remedies, virgin sugar pills are wetted with the desired liquid remedy and then allowed to dry. Alcohol (at least 70 percent) may be used for the last attenuation stage before wetting the pellets because water dissolves sugar too easily. The sugar may be lactose because it is less soluble than sucrose; sucrose can be used for lactose-intolerant patients. One drop of liquid remedy is used to medicate about forty ⅛-inch diameter pills.[15] Rice paper wafers can be used for patients who want to avoid all types of sugar, and glycerin is used for patients who want a liquid remedy but want to avoid alcohol.

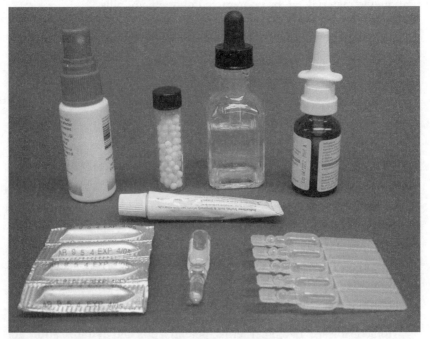

Figure 1.4. Some forms of homeopathic remedies. From left to right, starting with the back row: topical spray, sugar pills, water/alcohol liquid, nasal spray, ointment, suppositories, an ampoule for injections, and ophthalmic drops.

POTENCIES

Typical potencies for self-prescribing range up to 30X and 30C. Many professional homeopaths work primarily with 100C and higher remedies. Remedies up to 50,000C are common from many pharmacies, and custom remedies are available at almost any dilution, but the price goes up with the potency. Remedies up to 30X and 30C typically cost between five dollars and ten dollars for a few hundred pellets. The price for a small bottle of very high-potency remedies has a much wider range, roughly ten dollars to one hundred dollars, probably reflecting different manufacturing techniques. A 100,000C custom remedy costs over three thousand dollars from one manufacturer.[16] Remedies with potencies of 1,000,000C and higher have been used.

The higher cost of higher-potency remedies reflects the time it takes to do so many dilutions and successions. Allowing two minutes for each stage, a 1,000C remedy would take thirty-three hours to make. A 100,000C remedy would take one hundred times longer—about 3,300 hours of continuous work (figure 1.5). A 1,000,000C remedy would take about seventeen years, assuming eight hours of work per day and two hundred and fifty work days in a year. It is because of these impractically long times that other techniques are usually used to make very high potencies (see appendix 1).

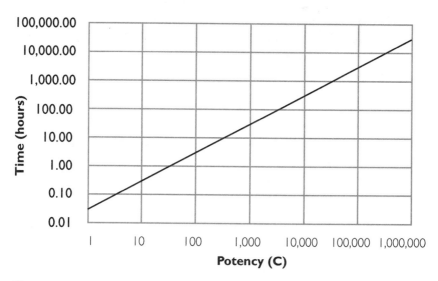

Figure 1.5. Estimate of remedy continues manufacturing time, assuming two minutes dillution/succussion.

Not all potencies are readily available or thought to be needed. Typical over-the-counter remedies for self-prescribing patients are 6, 12, and 30C and X. A typical professional set of remedies might contain 30C, 200C, 1,000C and 10,000C. Most in-between-strength remedies are not stocked because their effects are sufficiently close to those stocked that homeopaths do not feel they are needed.

IDENTIFYING AND CHARACTERIZING REMEDIES: PROVINGS

The data that determine which remedies may alleviate particular symptoms come from three sources. The dominant source and the most highly regarded (by homeopaths) is **provings** (also called **homeopathic pathogenetic trials** or HPTs). In provings (from the German *Pruefen*), healthy volunteers are given repeated doses of a remedy until symptoms start to appear. The volunteers then very carefully write down all their symptoms every day and often have daily consultations with their supervisors. The process continues until the symptoms seem to cease; typically this takes a few months. Different **provers** (participants) are thought to manifest symptoms related to different parts of the body, so the symptoms from all the provers are assembled into a composite picture of the remedy. Originally, provings used only low-potency and even **crude doses**, but Hahnemann soon switched to 30C remedies both for provings and for treating patients. Thus the very same remedy is believed to cause symptoms in healthy people and to cure patients with the same symptoms; proving reactions result from taking the remedy repeatedly, whereas healing is best stimulated by taking the remedy once or as few times as possible.

A second source of data comes from accidental poisonings by substances such as mercury and arsenic, which reveal some symptoms that these materials should be able to alleviate as homeopathic remedies.

The third source of data is from homeopaths' observations of their patients. If a symptom is seen to disappear when a sick person is treated with a particular remedy, then this symptom is considered a strong candidate for addition to the list of curable symptoms for that particular remedy.

MATERIA MEDICA

A carefully proved remedy will be found to cause hundreds of symptoms, and over a thousand in some cases. A **materia medica** is a book that lists the symptoms of each remedy. Reproduced below are the symptoms of Natrum muriaticum, according to noted homeopath William Boericke. Natrum muriaticum is sodium chloride, or common table salt. These are some of the symptoms that a homeopathic salt remedy is claimed to cause in healthy people, and hence to cure in sick people. The reader is not expected to study this quotation in detail but just to scan it for a sense of the number and nature of symptoms homeopathy associates with one of its remedies, and for how symptoms are usually organized. (Boericke's list of symptoms is relatively brief. Other references have many times more pages devoted to this remedy.)

Mind. Psychic causes of disease; ill effects of grief, fright, anger, etc. Depressed, particularly in chronic diseases. Consolation aggravates. Irritable; gets into a passion about trifles. Awkward, hasty. Wants to be alone to cry. Tears with laughter.

Head. Throbs. Blinding headache. Aches as if a thousand little hammers were knocking on the brain, in the morning on awakening, after menstruation, from sunrise to sunset. Feels too large; cold. Anemic headache of schoolgirls; nervous, discouraged, broken down. Chronic headache, semi-lateral, congestive, from sunrise to sunset, with pale face, nausea, vomiting; periodical; from eyestrain; menstrual. Before attack, numbness and tingling in lips, tongue and nose, relieved by sleep. Frontal sinus inflammation.

Eyes. Feel bruised, with headache in school children. Eyelids heavy. Muscles weak and stiff. Letters run together. Sees sparks. Fiery, zigzag appearance around all objects. Burning in eyes. Give out on reading or writing. Stricture of lachrymal duct with suppuration. Escape of muco-pus when pressing upon sac. Lachrymation, burning and acrid. Lids swollen. Eyes appear wet with tears. Tears stream down face on coughing. . . . Asthenapia due to insufficiency of internal recti muscles. . . . Pain in eyes when looking down. Cataract incipient. . . .

Ears. Noises, roaring and ringing.

Nose. Violent, fluent coryza, lasting from one to three days, then changing into stoppage of nose, making breathing difficult. Discharge thin and watery, like raw white of egg. Violent sneezing coryza. Infallible for stopping a cold commencing with sneezing. Use thirtieth potency. Loss of smell and taste. Internal soreness of nose. Dryness.

Face. Oily, shiny, as if greased. Earthy complexion. Fever-blisters. Mouth.—
Frothy coating on tongue, with bubbles on side. Sense of dryness.
Scorbutic gums. Numbness, tingling of tongue, lips, and nose. Vesicles and burning on tongue, as if there was a hair on it. Eruptions
around mouth and vesicles like pearls on lips. Lips and dowers of
mouth dry, ulcerated, and cracked. Deep crack in middle of lower lip.
Tongue mapped. . . . Loss of taste. Large vesicle on lower lip, which
is swollen and burns. Immoderate thirst.

Stomach. Hungry, yet loose flesh. . . . Heartburn, with palpitation. Un-
quenchable thirst. Sweats while eating. Craving for salt. Aversion to
bread, to anything slimy, like oysters; fats. Throbbing in pit. Sticking
sensation in cardiac orifice.

Abdomen. Cutting pain in abdomen. Distended. Pain in abdominal ring on
coughing.

Rectum. Burning pains and stitching after stool. Anus contracted, torn,
bleeding. Constipation; stool dry, crumbling. . . . Painless and
copious diarrhea, preceded by pinching pain in abdomen.

Urine. Pain just after urinating. . . . Increased, involuntary when walking,
coughing, etc. Has to wait a long time for it to pass if others are
present. . . .

Male. Emission, even after coitus. Impotence with retarded emission.

Female. Menses irregular; usually profuse. Vagina dry. Leucorrhoea acrid,
watery. Bearing-down pains; worse in morning. Prolapsus uteri, with
cutting in urethra. Ineffectual labor-pains. Suppressed menses. Hot
during menses.

Respiratory. Cough from a tickling in the pit of stomach, accompanied by
stitches in liver and spurting of urine. Stitches all over chest. Cough,
with bursting pain in head. Shortness of breath, especially on going
upstairs. Whooping-cough with flow of tears with cough.

Heart. Tachycardia. Sensation of coldness of heart. Heart and chest feel con-
stricted. Fluttering, palpitating; intermittent pulse. Heart's pulsations
shake body. Intermits on lying down.

Extremities. Pain in back, with desire for some firm support. Every movement
accelerates the circulation. Palms hot and perspiring. Arms and legs,
but especially knees, feel weak. Hangnails. Dryness and cracking
about finger-nails. Numbness and tingling in fingers and lower
extremities. Ankles weak and turn easily. Painful contraction of ham-
strings. Cracking in joints on motion. Coldness of legs with congestion to head, chest, and stomach.

Sleep. Sleepy in forenoon. Nervous jerking during sleep. Dreams of robbers.
Sleepless from grief.

Skin. Greasy, oily, especially on hairy parts. Dry eruptions, especially on
margin of hairy scalp and bends of joints. Fever blisters. Urticaria;

itch and burn. Crusty eruptions in bends of limbs, margin of scalp, behind ears. Warts on palms of hands. Eczema; raw, red, and inflamed; worse eating salt, at seashore. Affects hair follicles. Alopecia. Hives, itching after exertion. Greasy skin.

Fever. Chill between 9 and 11 A.M. Heat; violent thirst, increases with fever. Fever-blisters. Coldness of the body, and continued chilliness very marked. Hydraemia in chronic malarial states with weakness, constipation, loss of appetite, etc. Sweats on every exertion.

Modalities. Worse, noise, music, warm room, lying down; about 10 A.M., at seashore, mental exertion, consolation, heat, talking. Better, open air, cold bathing, going without regular meals, lying on right side; pressure against back, tight clothing.[17]

The **modalities** at the end of this list are the conditions believed to either aggravate or ameliorate all the previous symptoms. For instance, the symptoms tend to be worse in a noisy environment and at about 10 A.M., and the symptoms tend to wane when the patient is in open air or taking a cold bath. Modalities are an important part of a complete remedy description in homeopathy.

SELF-PRESCRIBING VERSUS CONSULTING A PROFESSIONAL HOMEOPATH

Many enthusiastic amateur homeopaths enjoy selecting remedies for themselves and their families and friends. However, homeopaths believe that an untrained amateur is less likely to find relief when self-prescribing than when a professional homeopath is involved. Nevertheless, many books encourage and help amateur homeopaths to self-prescribe, but most suggest treating only acute rather than chronic ailments.

A significant reason why professional help is thought to be less important for acute than for chronic conditions is that whole-person prescribing is believed to be less important in acute cases. Prescribing based mostly on the main physical complaints is believed to work for acute ailments; for example, Arnica is believed to be useful for bruising, bleeding, and pain resulting from falls or other accidents. Some homeopaths also recommend not exceeding potencies of 30X or 30C for self-prescribers in order to avoid the possibility of unpleasant reactions.

TAKING THE CASE

When a patient visits a homeopath, the homeopath "takes the **case**." Lab tests can be important in homeopathy; however, compared with conventional physicians, homeopaths rely more on patients' descriptions of their own symptoms.

A typical first visit usually lasts at least an hour. The homeopath is, of course, interested in why the patient came to see him, usually physical symptoms—what homeopaths call the **chief complaint**. The homeopath also needs details about the chief complaint, such as the color of nasal mucus when the patient has a cold or a detailed description of head pain if he or she has a headache. The homeopath will also want to know about all additional physical symptoms even though they may seem completely unrelated to the chief complaint, such as weak ankles or an unusual sleeping position if the chief complaint is headaches, or ringing in the ears if the chief complaint is a painful knee. Homeopaths call these simultaneous but seemingly unrelated symptoms **concomitants**.

The homeopath also needs to know the modalities of the symptoms: the factors that make the symptoms better or worse. These include conditions such as body position; movement of the body; weather; urination and defecation; sex; time of day; time of the year; phase of the moon; food and beverages; external stimuli such as noise, music, light and touch, rubbing, and conversation with others.

Homeopaths will usually also ask about the onset of the symptoms—when they started and whether their onset coincided with some event in the patient's life.

Homeopaths also need to know about one's **general symptoms**, or symptoms that do not affect just one part of the body. Examples are sluggishness, feelings of hot or cold, restless sleep, changes in appetite, and nervous energy.

Homeopaths particularly value what they call **strange, rare, and peculiar symptoms**. For instance, if a patient with a numbness feels better when lying on his back and pulling the hair in front of his ears,[18] his peculiar symptom points to a single remedy, Dioscorea.

Like physicians, homeopaths will usually want to know a patient's *medical history* and those of his or her parents and grandparents. It may also be relevant to know if anything traumatic or stressful happened to one's mother while she was pregnant.

All this is just the beginning because most homeopaths believe that *mental* and *emotional symptoms* are often the most important symptoms in a case. Homeopath Todd Rowe recommends the following questions to draw out these important symptoms:

> What do you love most about life?
>
> What concerns do others express about you?
>
> What are you teased most about?
>
> What bothers you the most about other people?
>
> What are you the most sensitive to?
>
> How do you feel about yourself?
>
> Where do you feel the most limited in your life?
>
> What don't you tell other people?
>
> How do you handle stress?
>
> What have been the most significant events in your life, and how did they affect you?[19]

Homeopaths may also use the patient's normal personality and appearance in selecting a remedy. For example, Pulsatilla may be effective for blonde women who are gentle and very emotional.

Physicians do not usually dig as deeply as homeopaths into the patient's personal life; they focus on identifying the illness or injury because that is what they treat. Homeopaths treat the whole person, especially in chronic cases, and hence need to know about the whole person before prescribing a remedy.

The complete notes from a thorough **case taking** are usually many pages long. From these, a homeopath will extract a summary. The following summary of a case involving uterine fibroids illustrates the common emphasis on nonphysical symptoms:

> Loquacious, loud
>
> Anxiety
>
> Doesn't want to live; desperate
>
> Feels humiliated, ashamed, used, rejected
>
> Angry, offended

Lonely

Religious affections

Workaholic, perfectionist, high level of achievement, success

Relationship problem, hard to get into the relationship

Absence of nurturing and love in childhood

High expectations of her from parents (mother)

Parents fighting (verbally and physically) with each other; threat of divorce

Alcoholism in the family

Fear of heights, of falling, of not being accepted

Uterine fibroids, lower abdomen swelling

Always hot

Constipated, retains fluids[20]

Based on such a summary, the homeopath will select the remedy.

REPERTORIES

A **repertory** has essentially the same information as a materia medica but reorganized. Materia medicae are organized by remedy; for each remedy, they list all the symptoms. Repertories are indexes to the remedies, organized by symptoms; for each symptom, they list all the remedies that cause and cure that symptom. With a list of a patient's symptoms, a homeopath can find in the repertory all the remedies that have ever caused each symptom in provings and hence might be a cure. Below is an extract from James Tyler Kent's *Repertory*; all the symptoms concern the patient's facial expression. The remedies are given as abbreviations of their Latin names. Facial expressions may not seem to be important symptoms for an illness, but all aspects of the patient are important to homeopathy because homeopathy treats the whole person. Again, the reader is not expected to study this extract in detail but just to scan it for a sense of the detailed nature of some of the symptoms and how a materia medica associates remedies with each symptom.

Facial Expression

anxious: Acon., aeth., agar., ail., all-c., aloe., am-c., am-m., ant-t., apis, ars., ars-h., bapt., bar-m., bell., bor., cact., calc., camph., canni., canth., carbo-o., carb-s., carb-v., chel., chin-a., chin.s., chlol., cic., coff., colch., coloc., crot-h., cupr., cupr-ar., cur., dig., dulc., eup-per., ferr-m., iris, kali-ar., kali-bi., kalm., lac-c., lat-m., lyc., lyss., merc., merc-c., morph., mygal., naja, nit-ac., nux-v., plb., sol-n., spig., spong., stram., stry., sulph., sul-ac., verat., vesp., vip., zinc.

anxious when child is lifted from cradle: Calc.

anxious during downward motion: Bor., gels.

astonished: Acon., bell., cann-s., carb-s., plb., stram.

besotted: Ail., bapt., bell., bry., bufo, cench., cocc., crot-c., crot-h., gels., lach., led., mur-ac., nux-m., op., sol-n., stram.

bewildered: Aesc., bry., carb-s., glon., lyc., nux-m., plb., stram., zinc.

cachectic: (See Sickly.)

changed: Aeth., ars., bufo, camph., caust., cham., colch., cupr., hell., ign., lyc., op., sec., squil., stram., verat.

childish: Anac., nux-m.

cold, distant: Puls.

confused: Aesc., ars., bufo, cupr-a., hyos., lyc., nat-m., phos., plb.

distressed: Ail., am-c., ars., aspar., cact., crot-l., cupr., iod., nux-m., nux-v., phos., stry., stram.

fierce: Bell., hydr-ac., merc-i-r., op.

foolish: Absin., acon., arg-n., bar-c., bufo, kali-br., lyc., phos., nux-m., stram.

frightened: Acon., apis, ars., atro., bapt., canth., cimic., cocc., kali-ar., lyss., sol-n., stram., stry., tab., tarent., vip., zinc.

frightened when aroused: Ail.

haggard: Am-c., ars., bell., camph., canth., caps., carb-v., colch., cupr., hydr., hyos., kali-ar., kali-c., kali-p., lach., merc., morph., naja, nat-m., nit-ac., op., ox-ac., phos., plb., sang., sec., sil., staph., stram., tab., verat-v.

happy: Apis, op.

idiotic: Agar., calc., kali-br., lach., laur., lyc., plb., sec., stram., tarent., thuj.

intoxicated: Bufo, cann-i., chlol., cocc., dor., eug., gels., hydr., hyos., kali-i., lach., led., merl., merc., mur-ac., nux-v., op., ruta, stram.

old looking: Abrot., ambr., arg-n., ars., ars-h., ars-i., aur-m., bar-c., calc., chlor., con., fl-ac., guaj., hydr-ac., iod., kreos., merc-c., nat-ma., ol-j., op., plb., sars., sep., staph., sulph.

old looking, sallow, wrinkled: Sep.

pinched: Acon., aeth., carb-an., carb-v., cina, cocc., cupr., ferr., iod., kali-n., merc., phos., sec., staph., tab., verat., verat-v., zinc.

sickly: Acon., aesc., aloe., alumn., anac., apis, arg-n., ars., ars-h., ars-i., berb., bism., bor., calc., calc-p., cann-i., carb-ac., carb-an., carb-s., carb-v., carl., caust., chel., chin., chin-s., cina, clem., cund., colch., con., cop., corn-c., crot-h., cupr., dig., eup-per., ferr., ferr-i., glon., gran., hura., iod., kali-ar., kali-bi., kali-c., kali-chl., kali-n., kali-p., kali-s., kreos., lach., lact., lyc., mag-m., mang., merc., naja, nat-m., nat-s., nit-ac., nux-m., nux-v., op., ph-ac., phos., plb., phyt., psor., ptel., rhus-t., sep., sil., spig., stann., staph., sulph., tab., tub., thuj., til., zinc.

sleepy: Cann-i., laur., nux-m., op., phos., phys.

stupid: Arg-n., arn., ars., ars-h., astar., bell., camph., cann-i., cann-s., chin-s., crot-c., cupr., ferr., gels., hell., hura, hydr., hyos., kali-br., lil-t., merc., nux-m., op., ox-ac., phos., phyt., plb., rhus-v., sec., stram., sulph., tab.

suffering: Acon., aeth., am-c., anac., ant-t., arg-n., ars., bor., cact., calc-ar., canth., carb-s., carb-v., caust., chel., chin-s., cocc., coloc., colch., cupr., helon., hyper., kali-ar., kali-br., kali-c., kali-p., kali-s., kreos., lach., lyss., mag-c., mag-m., mang., mez., nat-m., nit-ac., nux-m., ph-ac., phos., phyt., plat., plb., puls., raph., sec., sil., stry., stram., sulph., sul-ac.

sullen: Alum., nux-v.

tired: Acon., ars., cimic., stram.

vacant: Anac., anan., bell., camph., carb-s., cic., cocc., ferr., hell., hyos., kali-br., lac., mez., op., ph-ac., stram., zinc. . . .[21]

Most repertories are organized primarily by parts of the body, and within each broad category, symptoms are arranged alphabetically. The intent is to make it easy to look up the symptoms and find the corresponding remedies.

The symptoms listed in a repertory are called **rubrics**. Symptoms that emerge from new provings usually fit existing rubrics, but sometimes new rubrics must be created because a symptom is new to homeopathy.

SELECTING THE REMEDY: THE SIMILLIMUM

The objective in remedy selection is to get the best match between the patient's symptoms and the symptoms caused by the remedy. Homeopaths select a small number of the symptoms, as in the case summary for the uterine fibroid patient quoted previously—the ones they believe are the most critical and most likely to highlight a single remedy. Special value is placed on **characteristic symptoms**, symptoms that are relatively rare, strange, or peculiar, and hence tend to distinguish the patient from others with the same chief complaint. Each symptom needs to be known in its "totality," which typically includes its location, its detailed description, and its modalities. The homeopath then looks up each symptom in a repertory, notes all the remedies that have caused that symptom, and then determines which remedies are involved most often. In theory, if one remedy is associated with all the symptoms and no other remedy is associated with more than half of the symptoms, then this remedy is thought to be the right one. In practice, it is never so clear. In any case, the final step is always to read the complete **symptom picture** of the remedy in a materia medica to make sure that it fits the patient's symptom picture. The remedy whose symptom picture best matches the patient's symptoms is the simillimum and hence should cure the patient. It is important that some of the patient's key symptoms be included in the remedy, but they need not all be included. It also does not matter that the remedy usually covers many more symptoms than the patient has.

A consequence of taking into account all the patient's symptoms is that different patients with the same chief complaints usually get different remedies. An online source gives the following example:

> [T]wo toddlers with ear infections may have similar symptoms but one may be weepy and clingy, wanting to sit in her mother's lap for kisses, hugs and consolation, while the other may be cranky and irritable, demanding toys or food and then throwing the requested object on the floor, to the mother's despair. The first child would be given Pulsatilla, the latter Chamomila.[22]

Another homeopath states: "Theoretically there should be as many types of pneumonia as there are people who have it,"[23] and thus each pneumonia patient might get a different remedy; homeopathic remedies are individualized. Similarly, most remedies are useful for treating a wide variety of primary complaints.

The amount of data in repertories and materia medicae is so staggering that use of computers is increasingly common. The remedy Sulphur has 12,384 rubrics (symptoms) listed in the Synthesis repertory,[24] and the total number of rubrics in the repertory is over 129,000.

FOLLOW-UP

Patients do not always get well immediately after taking a remedy. Follow-up consultations with the homeopath are often needed. The homeopath will reassess the case, sometimes by phone, usually in much less time than the initial visit took. The homeopath may then ask the patient just to continue waiting for the remedy to act, may suggest additional doses or a different potency of the same remedy, or may prescribe an entirely different remedy. For chronic health problems it can take weeks, months, and even many years to find an apparently effective remedy or series of remedies.

THEORY OF HUMAN HEALTH: THE VITAL FORCE

Homeopaths believe that we all have a vital force, a nonphysical entity that is the essence of life (it leaves when we die) and that strives to keep us in good health. Hahnemann described the vital force as follows:

> In the state of health the spirit-like vital force (*dynamis*) animating the material human organism reigns in supreme sovereignty. It maintains the sensations and activities of all the parts of the living organism in a harmony that obliges wonderment. The reasoning spirit who inhabits the organism can thus freely use this healthy living instrument to reach the lofty goal of human existence.[25]

If the vital force is disturbed, deranged, or out of balance, the person becomes ill. The vital force responds by producing symptoms. The symptoms reveal how our bodies are coping with the assault; the symptoms are the evidence that our vital force is trying to get back in balance. Examples of such symptoms are sweating when we are hot and vomiting in response to food poisoning. In these examples, the reason for the body's reaction is clear. Homeopaths believe that *all* symptoms serve such purposes, even though in most cases we may not understand the root imbalance of the vital force or how the particular symptoms help to correct the imbalance. In this view, medications that merely alleviate symptoms offer only temporary relief and are not very helpful. Permanent relief will follow only if the vital force is rebalanced. Our symptoms are our bodies' attempt to fight the sickness and thus should be honored rather than suppressed.

Homeopathic remedies do not fight the disease itself; rather, they are thought to stimulate the vital force "by calming its excesses and strengthening its deficiencies,"[26] so that it can fight the illness. Homeopathic remedies are also thought to help prevent illnesses by strengthening the vital force when it is not out of balance.

THE VITAL FORCE: A CONTROVERSIAL CONCEPT

It is instructive to read Hahnemann's description of how the vital force (life force in this translation) cures:

> The life force, that glorious power innate in the human being, was ordained to conduct life in the most perfect way *during its health.* The life force, which is equally present in all parts of the organism (in the sensible as well as the irritable fiber) is the untiring mainspring of all normal natural bodily functions. It was not at all created for the purpose of helping itself in diseases....

1. True medical art is that cogitative pursuit which devolves upon the higher human spirit, free deliberation, and the selecting intellect which decides according to well-founded reasons.
2. It does so in order to differently tune the instinctual (intellect- and awareness-lacking) automatic and energic [sic] life force when the life force has been mistuned, through disease, to abnormal activity.
3. It differently tunes the life force by means of an affection similar to that of the disease, engendered by a medicine that has been homeopathically selected.
4. By means of this medicine, the life force is rendered medicinally sick to such a degree (in fact a somewhat higher degree) that the natural affection can no longer work on the life force.
5. In this way, the life force becomes rid of the natural disease, remaining occupied solely with the so similar, somewhat stronger medicinal disease-affection against which the life force now directs its whole energy and which it soon overcomes.
6. The life force thereby becomes free and able again to return to the norm of health and to its actual intended purpose: that of enlivening and sustaining the healthy organism.
7. It can do this without having suffered painful or debilitating attacks by this transformation.[27]

Hahnemann's intended meaning is not entirely clear. Noted homeopath Luc De Schepper explains:

> The remedy thus produces a stronger disease picture, expelling the

similar weaker illness, according to Nature's Law: "Two similar diseases cure each other." The Vital Force is freed now from the influence of the natural disease, while the influence of the remedy is transient because of its minuteness. Soon the Vital Force becomes free of the influence of the artificial disease too, leading to a cure.[28]

Even with this explanation, the concept of the vital force is difficult to grasp. Anthony Campbell, a physician with extensive practical experience in complementary/alternative medicine, bluntly appraises "energy" healing and the vital force:

> The "energy" that practitioners of alternative medicine often speak about is closely related to vitalism. *Like the vital force*, it doesn't have any identifiable source, it doesn't obey any kind of law, it can't be defined. It is simply postulated ad hoc, to explain whatever effects or alleged effects needs [sic] explaining. It can't be pinned down or put to the question; its function is to provide the illusion of meaning without the substance. It is a little like the ether which was postulated in earlier times to explain the transmission of light through space, or like phlogiston, which was used at one time to explain the phenomenon of heat. . . . However, phlogiston and the ether could be, and were, disproved by experiment, so at least they were open to disproof and so were scientific theories; "energy" in alternative medicine can't be disproved because it is too amorphous and vague a concept.[29]
>
> Historically, the vital force has been controversial within homeopathy. Some practitioners, such as British homeopath Richard Hughes (1836–1902), rejected some of the more ethereal aspects of homeopathy, namely the vital force, miasm theory (see chapter 7), and homeopathy's nonmolecular remedies (see chapter 3). During the battles between various factions over a century ago, one homeopath commented on the vital force: "Such a preposterous doctrine will not bear the touch of exact science for a moment. It is only a relic of the old metaphysical system of philosophizing, which accepted a name in lieu of an explanation."[30]
>
> The vital force has no directly observable properties. It is a theoretical construct formulated to try to explain health and illness and is clearly not today's best explanation.[31] Most homeopaths ignore the vastly improved understanding of biochemistry, pathogens and genetics that has come in the last two centuries.

Interestingly, the vital force does not guide core homeopathic practice; remedies are selected on the basis of the Law of Similars, not the vital force. Hahnemann himself made no use of the vital force until the later editions of his *Organon*. "In the early editions," Campbell notes, "he was if anything dismissive of the idea."[32] Most homeopaths' continuing belief in the vital force is difficult for many outsiders to understand.

NOTES

1. David Sollars, *The Complete Idiot's Guide to Homeopathy* (Indianapolis: Alpha Books, 2002), p. 45.

2. R. U. Ramakrishnan and Catherine R. Coulter, *A Homeopathic Approach to Cancer* (St. Louis: Quality Medical Publishing, 2001), p. 76.

3. Samuel Hahnemann, Aphorism 273, *Organon of the Medical Art*, 6th ed., edited and annotated by Wenda O'Reilly (Redmond, Wash.: Birdcage Books, 1996). Italics in original.

4. Julian Winston, *The Faces of Homeopathy* (New Zealand: Great Auk Publishing, 1999), p. 505. Some controversy remains about the origin of succussion. It may originally have been just a way of assuring thorough mixing. However, Hahnemann (and other early homeopaths such as Francis E. Boericke) expressed concern that the potency of liquid medicines carried by practitioners who traveled by horse would become excessively potent due to the jostling.

5. Many of these examples, including the quotation, are from Robert Ullman and Judyth Reichenberg-Ullman, *The Patient's Guide to Homeopathic Medicine* (Edmonds, Wash.: Picnic Point Press, 1995).

6. Some homeopaths believe that a symptom can be useful for selecting the remedy but will not go away when the remedy is taken.

7. *The Homeopathic Pharmacopoeia of the United States, Abstracts: 2001* (Washington, D.C.: Homoeopathic Pharmacopoeia Convention of the United States, 2001). Hereafter HPUS.

8. Constantine Hering, quoted in Steven Kayne, *Homeopathic Pharmacy* (New York: Churchill Livingston, 1997), p. 101.

9. Jeremy Sherr, *Dynamic Provings*, vol. 1 (Malvern, U.K.: Dynamis Books, 1997), p. 125.

10. Hering, p. 46.

11. Some pharmacists consider the mother tincture to be 0X, but the HPUS says it is 1X.

12. The primary potential difference between an attenuation and the corresponding liquid remedy is the solvent. For attenuations, the solvent is usually

water. For most liquid remedies, the solvent is about 20 percent alcohol in water, which is achieved by using this alcohol and water combination for the last dilution.

13. Curiously, according to the HPUS, making centesimal remedies starts with making 1X and then 2X attenuations. This 2X attenuation is then called a 1C attenuation, and subsequent attenuations all involve dilutions of a factor of one hundred.

14. Miranda Castro, *The Complete Homeopathy Handbook* (New York: St. Martin's Press, 1990), p. 13. This solubility assumption is curious. An insoluble material cannot be made soluble by any amount of mortar-and-pestle grinding. Grinding can shorten the *time* it takes to dissolve as much of the material as can dissolve, but it does not change the *amount* that can dissolve. However, grinding and dilution may result in the absence of pieces of the original material that are visible to the naked eye. The view that the material was completely dissolved was perhaps reasonable two hundred years ago when homeopathy was invented.

15. HPUS, p. 44.

16. Hahnemann Labs [online], "Custom Remedies," http://www.hahnemannlabs.com/custom_remedy_preparation.html [May 5, 2002].

17. William Boericke, *Materia Medica with Repertory,* 9th ed. (Santa Rosa, Calif.: Boericke and Tafel, 1927), pp. 368–70. The 1927 date of this publication causes no loss of reputability; in fact, many homeopaths put more faith in older books than in more recent publications.

18. Timothy F. Allen, "Dioscorea" in *The Encyclopedia of Pure Materia Medica* [online], http://www.homeoint.org/allen/d/dios-8.htm [July 6, 2002].

19. Todd Rowe, *Homeopathic Methodology* (Berkeley: North Atlantic Books, 1998), p. 8.

20. A. Y. Popen, "A Case of Uterine Fibroids," *Simillimum* 14, no. 1 (2001): 56.

21. James Tyler Kent, *Repertory of the Homeopathic Materia Medica* (1897–1899; reprint, New Delhi: B. Jain Publishers, 1998), pp. 374–75.

22. B. Lennihan and J. Riedlinger, "An Introduction to Homeopathy, Part 2," [online], http://www.altcorp.com/homeopathy.htm [Nov. 17, 2002].

23. Elizabeth Wright-Hubbard, *A Brief Study Course in Homeopathy* (St. Louis: Formur, 1997), p. 5.

24. *Synthesis Eight for Radar* (Assesse, Belgium: Archibel, 2002).

25. Samuel Hahnemann, Aphorism 9, *Organon of the Medical Art*, 6th ed., translated by Künzli, Naudé, and Pendleton (Blaine, Wash.: Cooper Publishing, 1982).

26. Richard Moskowitz, *Resonance: The Homeopathic Point of View* http://www.Xlibris.com (Xlibris Corporation, 2000), p. 28.

27. Wenda O'Reilly, Introduction, Samuel Hahnemann, *Organon of the Medical Art*, 6th ed., edited and annotated by Wenda O'Reilly (Redmond, Wash.: Birdcage Books, 1996), pp. 37–38.

28. Luc De Schepper, *Hahnemann Revisited* (Santa Fe: Full of Life Publishing, 2001), p. 28.

29. Anthony Campbell, "Key Ideas in Alternative Medicine" [online], http://homepage.ntlworld.com/anthony.campbell1/essays/altmed/keyideas.html [March 2, 2002].

30. Originally published in 1883–84 and quoted in Harris Coulter, *Divided Legacy* (Berkeley: North Atlantic Books, 1982), p. 357.

31. This is, of course, a scientific perspective. Properties of "good" theories are explained in chapter 9, and in that context the weakness of the vital force theory becomes clear.

32. Anthony Campbell, *Homeopathy in Perspective,* [online], http://www.accampbell.uklinux.net/homeopathy/index.html [March 11, 2002], chap. 3.

2. Types of Homeopathy:
Commonalities and Contradictions

There are many different schools of and practices in homeopathy. Many homeopaths feel that all of them work and that this diversity is a demonstration of the pervasive power and continuing growth of homeopathy. Others do not doubt the effectiveness of the various approaches but believe that many of them should not be called *homeopathy* because they do not follow Hahnemann's principles. Still others believe that the issue is not just one of naming but of effectiveness; they feel that some of the non-classical approaches have not been adequately tested and hence may not work, or not work as well as classical homeopathy. The controversies surrounding this topic come from within homeopathy, not from the outside.[1] Hence, no matter how the various so-called homeopathic practices are classified, some homeopaths will disagree with the classification.

This variety of practices all labeled as "homeopathy" means that everyone can find something to criticize. The same diversity of practices also invites an answer to such criticism: "Your criticism is not valid because what you criticized is not *real* homeopathy." In reality, there is no clear place to draw the line.

Classical homeopathy was described in chapter 1. Other approaches to homeopathy are emphasized in this chapter and arranged in approximate decreasing order of prominence in homeopathic literature. This chapter also includes a critical look at three issues: the doctrine of signatures, single versus combination remedies, and the longevity of controversies within homeopathy.

MAJOR TYPES OF HOMEOPATHY

Most homeopaths consider the following practices to be part of homeopathy. This consensus is exemplified by the explanation of these practices in most books on homeopathy and their inclusion in **meta-analyses** of clinical trials.

As explained in chapter 1, in classical homeopathy, the remedy is based on all the patient's symptoms, and only a single remedy is used at a time. Virtually any patient complaint can be treated, not just standard physical ailments. Provings are the primary source of the data for determining what the remedy can cure. Mental symptoms are often considered very important. Some self-declared purists would say that only classical homeopathy should be defined as homeopathy.

In **clinical homeopathy**, a single remedy (usually) is prescribed based on a diagnosed illness or single symptom, as in **conventional medicine**, not on the whole person. The European American Coalition on Homeopathy explains: "In clinical homeopathy, the selection of the medication is based on the chief clinical symptoms of the illness to be treated. . . . Here, the 'Similar' concept relates above all to the local and/or acute syndromes displayed by the patient."[2]

Combination homeopathy (or **complex homeopathy**) uses *formula remedies*, which are standard mixtures of many remedies, all of which treat the same symptom or group of related symptoms. For instance, a headache combination might contain a mixture of eight remedies, each of which includes headaches as one of its symptoms. Such remedies are very popular as over-the-counter remedies. Using remedy mixtures is also sometimes called *homeotherapeutics*. Obviously, combination remedies are not individualized.

In **isopathy**, remedies are made from the agents that cause the condition being treated. A person allergic to cats might be given a cat-hair-based remedy; amalgam remedies are used to treat symptoms thought to come from amalgam (mercury alloy) fillings. Isopathy has nothing to do with matching symptoms and hence provings of remedies are not needed; it does not treat the whole person and hence there is no individualization of remedies. In isopathy, the external cause of the illness is presumed to be known, whereas in classical homeopathy, substantive external causes such as bacteria and viruses are irrelevant; it is the symptoms that are treated, not an identifiable disease. In isopathy, "same cures same;" in homeopathy, "like cures like."

LESS COMMON PRACTICES ASSOCIATED WITH HOMEOPATHY

The following practices are mentioned in some homeopathy books but have not been evaluated significantly in clinical trials.

Homeopathic immunology or *homeopathic prophylaxis* is used by homeopaths who believe that remedies prevent particular illnesses; clearly, such prescriptions cannot be based on an individual's symptoms. Homeopathic disease prevention is discussed in chapter 12.

When practitioners want to alleviate the side effects of conventional medicines, they sometimes use **tautopathy**: treating a patient taking a conventional drug with a homeopathically prepared (diluted and succussed), remedy made from the same drug to reduce or eliminate the side effects of the full-strength conventional medicine. Thus, a high-potency chemotherapy remedy might be used to treat side effects of chemotherapy. (Homeopathy does not explain why the remedy only counters the undesirable side effects and not the intentional curative effects of the conventional drugs.) Another variation of tautopathy is the use of potentized homeopathic remedies to counteract the desire for the material itself. For example, a patient suffering from chocolate addiction might be given potentized chocolate.[3]

Some homeopaths ignore any proving or toxicological data in selecting remedies. An example is the use of the ancient **doctrine of signatures**. An advocate of this doctrine, the medieval alchemist Paracelsus, wrote, "God would not place a disease upon the Earth without providing a cure for it, and a clue to the cure's identity. He places a signature upon it by making remedies resemble the organs or maladies they can cure."[4] According to this view, if the patient has kidney problems, a kidney bean might work because of the similarity of its shape to that of kidneys. Since Arnica grows near mountains, it must be a good remedy for bruises from falls. Remedies made from creeping plants are thought to help cure desire for or dreams of travel. Plants with profuse milky juice (such as euphorbia) should increase milk production in nursing mothers. Walnuts are supposed to be good for head ailments since the nutmeat resembles a small brain.

In a contrasting approach, *constitutional prescribing*, the homeopath bases the prescription on the general characteristics, or **constitution** of the healthy patient, consisting of personality and physical characteristics.[5] When **constitutional remedies** are used on a sick patient, the symptoms of the patient's illness are ignored. When used on a well patient, constitutional prescribing is supposed to increase the patient's resistance to getting sick.

Bach flower remedies (flower essences) are sometimes perceived as part of homeopathy; the *British Homeopathic Pharmacopoeia* has specifications for their preparation, and the popular Rescue Remedy is incorrectly thought to be homeopathic by most of its users; it is a Bach flower remedy. However, Bach flower remedies are not potentized—no succussion accompanies the dilution, and there are no provings as a guide to prescribing, so the Law of Similars is not involved in their application. Edward Bach (1886–1936) discovered the power of flowers. Steven Kayne notes: "If he [Bach] experienced a sudden adverse emotion and went outside to seek fresh air and exercise, he would always be drawn inextricably toward a particular plant or tree. Simply being in its presence would relieve his emotional state. He believed . . . he had been led divinely towards a new method of healing."[6]

THE DOCTRINE OF SIGNATURES

Many classical homeopaths disdain the doctrine of signatures in favor of what they believe to be evidence-based remedies, founded primarily on provings. Hahnemann himself opposed the doctrine of signatures because it was not evidence-based. Nonetheless, the doctrine maintains a strong presence in homeopathy, as evidenced by the following three factors.

1. Most published provings have long introductions about the tested substance, including its history, its properties, and its role in society. This approach is unique to homeopathy; published papers in conventional science rarely give this kind of information. The difference suggests that this information is important to homeopathy: There is a strong expectation among homeopaths that the remedy's healing properties will have something to do with its anatomical, cultural, technical, and historic aspects.
2. Some homeopaths feel that they can make good predictions about the usefulness of a remedy before proving it: Jeremy Sherr comments,

"Before making my final choice on a proving remedy I always meditate on the key questions: Will this remedy be a useful tool in
restoring the sick to health? Will this remedy fill a gap that homeopaths encounter in their daily practice?"[7] It certainly would be useful
to know the answers to these questions before going to the trouble
of conducting a proving, but how can the experimenter know anything about these issues in advance? How does one meditate on the
probable usefulness of diamond and neon? The only way is by using
the doctrine of signatures—speculating about the physical, chemical,
historical, or economic aspects of the substance for clues as to its
healing capabilities.

3. Some homeopaths use the doctrine of signatures outright, believing
that a plant with an eyelike pattern on its leaves should be useful as
an eye remedy.

Specific homeopathic applications of the doctrine of signatures raise
questions about the doctrine's validity:

- Since the thorn apple grows in cemeteries, homeopaths believe it is
an effective remedy (Stramonium) for people who fear cemeteries.[8]
But why pick on this one plant, given that there are hundreds of
others that grow in cemeteries, particularly if one looks worldwide?
And why is it not the remedy for obsession for cemeteries, or for
people who work in cemeteries?

- When his patient's behavior reminded a particular homeopath of
mosquitoes, the mosquito remedy (Culex musca) was given.[9] Yet
there are many flighty and annoying insects. It is difficult to distinguish
among mosquito-, fly-, gnat-, wasp-, and beelike behavior in people,
and hence difficult for such behavior to point to a unique remedy
derived from a specific insect.

- A boy who acted like a cat was given Lac felinum (cat's milk remedy).
Why cat's *milk*? Why not cat hair, blood, or urine?

- Some homeopaths believe that tea remedy (thea) will cure illness in
people who are obsessed with collecting tea sets. But might not the
hobby of collecting tea sets be just coincidental to the patient's illness?[10]

- Aurum (gold) is said to be effective for people with depression and
low self-esteem because gold is so valuable. Platina (platinum) is said
to be good for haughty people because platinum is such a rare element. Note the inconsistency in that gold treats an opposite; platinum
treats a similar.[11]

If the doctrine of signatures has no validity, how can the existence of provings symptoms that resemble the original material be explained? (1) Each starting material has dozens of properties with hundreds of interpretations, and most remedies have either hundreds or thousands of symptoms; thus it is always possible in retrospect to find some coincidences. This makes the doctrine of signatures *feel* like it works, but also may make it untestable due to lack of falsifiability (chapter 9). (2) In a few provings, the provers know what is being proved. In most provings, those doing the data extraction know what is being proved. Hence the expectations of provers and researchers may influence their findings.

Although many homeopaths embrace and use the doctrine of signatures, many others do not: Homeopath Karl Robinson, M.D., does not mince his words: "As for the Doctrine of Signatures? Rubbish. Unfettered balderdash."[12] As is often the case, homeopaths do not agree with one another.

PERIPHERAL TECHNIQUES IN HOMEOPATHY

In addition to the various schools of homeopathy, many of which deviate from Hahnemann's teachings, a number of techniques for selecting remedies are even further removed. For instance, some homeopaths use **dowsing** for diagnosis and to select the appropriate remedy. The dowsing tool is usually a small, handheld pendulum. For selecting the remedy, the pendulum is held over each of the candidate bottles (figure 2.1); the pattern of the supposedly spontaneous swinging indicates whether it is the correct remedy; for some practitioners, clockwise indicates yes and counterclockwise indicates no. This method is sometimes used in conjunction with classical homeopathy after the remedy selection has been narrowed down to a few possibilities. This approach seems to assume some sixth sense or psychic ability on the part of the practitioner.

Another reasonably common technique, **applied kinesiology**, involves muscle strength testing. In one form, the patient holds a proposed remedy in one hand and raises an arm to a horizontal position. The practitioner then tries to push the arm down while the patient resists (figure 2.2). The claim is that the patient's resistance will be stronger when holding the correct remedy. In another form, the patient's thumb and a finger form an *O*. The practitioner tests the force needed to break the O. Besides being used to select homeopathic remedies, this technique and dowsing are sometimes used to select many other types of remedies and dietary supplements.

Less common is the use of *iridology*, the belief that everything about the health of a person is revealed by looking at his or her eyes. In this view, the detailed patterns and colors of the patient's irises can be used to diagnose the health of the body, as well as inherited susceptibilities, and thus can be used to help select the homeopathic remedy.

Electrodiagnostics, the use of electronic devices to select the appropriate homeopathic remedy, is attractive to some practitioners and patients. Some devices measure electrical resistance of the body, for

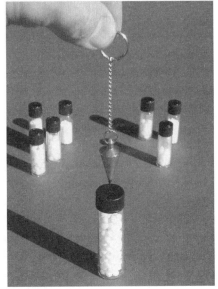

Figure 2.1. Dowsing with a pendulum to select the correct remedy.

instance between acupuncture points. Remedies are prescribed to correct any detected "imbalances." In some cases, measurements are made while the patient holds candidate remedies or while the bottled remedy is placed on the electronic circuit; the electrical response indicates whether the remedy is appropriate. Other devices claim to match the "resonance" of the remedy to that of the disease.

None of these techniques is supported in Hahnemann's writings. Although they fit the New Age worldview, scientists and engineers tend to discount all of homeopathy by association because they believe at least these peripheral techniques cannot be valid.

Consistency testing of some of these peripheral techniques would be a simple and valuable first step in determining whether they work. For instance, does a practitioner of applied kinesiology get the same results when the technique is repeated in double-blind experiments (with neither the practitioner nor the patient knowing which remedy is being tested)? Do different practitioners get the same results for the same case in double-blind testing? I had an opportunity in 2001 to do some informal testing with a practitioner who used dowsing with a small pendulum. We conducted three series of tests for consistency, to see whether the practitioner selected the same remedy in repeated trials. The results were negative.

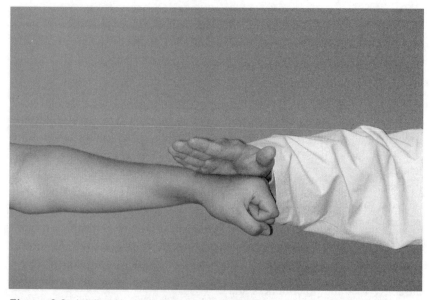

Figure 2.2. Applied kinesiology for remedy selection.

Because the homeopathic application of these techniques has not been given much serious attention by researchers, there is little hard evidence on their effectiveness. However, many of these techniques have been tested in other contexts; dowsing for water and applied kinesiology and iridology for diagnosing health problems have all been found ineffective in controlled scientific testing.[13]

COMBINATION VERSUS SINGLE REMEDIES

Remedy mixtures are clearly aimed at a particular ailment or disease, as indicated by their names: Depression, Sore Throat, Earache, Teething, Constipation, Body Pure, Anxiety, Flu, Arthritis, Acne, Headache, No Jet-Lag, and SnoreStop. An advertisement in *Homeopathy Today* states: "The plan is that one of the remedies will be near enough the simillimum to trigger the right healing response in a variety of cases, while the others will be generally ignored."[14]

Certainly one reason for the popularity of combination remedies is that it is so obvious which one to use; no training is needed. The clear association of a remedy with a symptom or disease also mirrors conventional medicine, perhaps making the process more comfortable for some patients.

Combination remedies are inconsistent with classical homeopathy in a number of ways: In classical homeopathy, (1) the chief complaint is often the least important symptom when selecting the simillimum; (2) almost all of the remedies in a mixture are incorrect (not the simillimum), and repeated doses of an incorrect remedy can result in an inadvertent proving; (3) some remedies are believed to antidote other remedies; therefore, even if the right remedy is in the mix, one of the other remedies in the mix may prevent it from working; and (4) Hahnemann instructed his followers to use only one remedy at a time.[15]

Classically there is nothing inherently wrong in having many different compounds in a remedy; for example, most remedies made from plants start with the hundreds of different chemical compounds that plants naturally contain. The difference is that these particular combinations have been proven. Mixed remedies could work, but each combination needs to be proved first. To be true to classical homeopathy, the proved mixture would be prescribed based on the complete symptoms picture. Thus, there still would not be one remedy that would relieve most headaches.

Homeopaths are not in agreement on combination homeopathy. Many believe combination remedies are useful, but others do not. Elizabeth Wright-Hubbard states bluntly: "Some mongrel homeopaths when in doubt give mixed prescriptions."[16]

Bill Gray states more tactfully: "Combination remedies may work on occasion, but more often than not they sell because the complaint is self-limited in the first place. Homeopathic understanding is that once remedies are mixed together, the resultant vibration is not identical to the sum of the separate parts. It becomes an entity of its own, which may or may not work in a given case. The analogy here is like trying to enhance a musical experience by mixing together all six of Bach's Brandenburg concertos all at the same time."[17]

COMMONALITIES AND DISCUSSION

The primary commonality among most of the above schools and techniques is the belief that dilution and succussion result in useful remedies.

Which practices can most legitimately be classified as homeopathy? If the single criterion is use of the Law of Similars, the foundation of homeopathy, then classical, clinical, and combination homeopathy all make the grade, but isopathy, tautopathy, immunology, the doctrine of signatures, dowsing, kinesiology, electrodiagnosis, iridology, and Bach flower remedies do not. If treating the whole person and individualization are added, then only classical homeopathy fits the definition.

Even classical homeopathy is hard to define. For some practitioners, the term means Hahnemann's homeopathy; for others, the central figure is James Tyler Kent (1849–1916), a renowned American homeopath. Compared with Hahnemann, Kent tended to use higher potencies, was a stronger advocate of constitutional prescribing, and put more emphasis on mental symptoms. Kent and all other homeopaths of his time were unaware of Hahnemann's latest ideas, such as **LM** remedies (see appendix 1), because Hahnemann's final edition of the *Organon* was not published until 1921. Even those who dismiss Kent and believe that Hahnemann alone represents the true path argue with one another over what Hahnemann meant in his writings. Thus an agreed-on definition of classical homeopathy does not exist.

Many practitioners cite the writings of Hahnemann to support their preferred variety of homeopathy. Another group of nominally classical homeopaths argues that Hahnemann could have been wrong in some respects or that his work may have been incomplete. This second group contends that homeopathy should not be stagnant and that new methods have been and continue to be developed and should be accepted if they are effective , just as they are in conventional medicine.

WHY ARE CONTROVERSIES WITHIN HOMEOPATHY SO INTENSE AND LONG-LIVED?

Homeopathy has always been torn by dissension. Historically, much of the debate centered on high versus low potencies, **miasms** (chapter 7), and the vital force. Today practitioners disagree about some newer ways of selecting the appropriate remedy. Classical homeopaths argue with the moderns over who is practicing "real" homeopathy. When asked if he would invite modern homeopath Rajan Sankaran to his school, classical homeopath George Vithoulkas was characteristically outspoken: "If he goes back to real things, yes. However, not if he continues like this. Sankaran alone has done more harm to homeopathy than all the enemies of homeopathy together. And [Jan] Scholten. These two especially, with the nonsense they circulate."[18]

A relatively tame response to criticism of the moderns is the following letter to the editor of *Homeopathy Today*:

Dear Editor:

It was with a heavy heart that we read the latest edition *of Homeopathy Today*. The editorial attacks on the ideas of Rajan Sankaran, Jan Scholten, Nancy Herrick, Todd Rowe and others are unwarranted. While it is very clear that Mr. Winston [editor of *Homeopathy Today*] has a great love for and desire to protect homeopathy, his sweeping use of the editorial position to advocate his personal beliefs has become a detriment to the National Center [for Homeopathy]. Many people have dropped their membership in the NCH because of the increasingly divisive tone in the newsletter. No good to homeopathy can come from one person or group trying to impose their idea of what is "good homeopathy" upon others. Let ideas and clinical results speak for themselves. Thus this letter has been examined, co-edited, and co-signed by a large number of concerned and prominent homeopaths who wish to raise their voices against intolerance and divisiveness. We have much important work ahead of us; we cannot allow ourselves to be sidetracked by partisan bickering.[19]

Conventional sciences like geology, physics, medicine, and biology also have intense debates, but with two important differences. (1) The debates among conventional scientists rarely concern the definition of the field itself. Geologists do not argue over what geology is and who is doing real geology but whether an asteroid impact or some other phenomenon caused the dinosaurs to become extinct. (2) Most disagreements in conventional sciences are eventually resolved and the field moves on to new challenges.

Many of homeopathy's debates have been going on for a century and a half and many will continue indefinitely. They are rarely resolved for four primary reasons. (1) An important technique whereby traditional science tends to avoid endless controversy is through asking only questions that can be resolved by experiments and observations. Who has the best dog? Is there a God? and What is beyond the detectable universe? are questions that cannot be answered by experiments and hence are not considered part of science. Homeopaths have no hesitancy in wrestling with questions that have little likelihood of being resolved through experiments. (2) One way homeopaths try to win debates is by quoting Hahnemann. Unfortunately, Hahnemann was not the clearest of writers,[20] he changed his mind on many issues, and most people read his works in translation from the original German. An entire book has recently been published claiming that all the standard translations of Hahnemann's *Organon* are misleading and consequently almost no one is practicing true Hahnemannian homeopathy.[21] These debates will never end because we cannot ask Hahnemann to clarify what he meant. (3) Homeopathy, unlike science, has no universally accepted and high-quality method for conducting experiments. The vast majority of homeopaths rely on their personal observations. (4) There is a dearth of funding to conduct the quality research which might resolve some of the controversies. Together, these last two factors may result in decades going by without resolution of controversies that are capable of being answered empirically.

At present, all the schools of homeopathy seem to be thriving despite their inconsistencies, and testing done to date has not revealed significant differences in cure rates. Since different approaches will usually result in different remedies for the same patient, the fact that so many of the approaches seem to be equally successful suggests that the particular choice of remedy may not be critical.

The remainder of this book focuses primarily on classical homeopathy. Despite the fact that even homeopaths do not agree on all the details of what classical homeopathy is, it is the least controversial form of homeopathy.

NOTES

1. See, for example, John Lunstroth, "It's Time for a Clear Definition of Homeopathy," *Homeopathy Today* 21, no. 8 (2001): 28–29.

2. European American Coalition on Homeopathy (EACH), *Homeotherapy: Definitions and Therapeutic Schools* (Huningue, France: Editions Medico-Pharmaceutiques Raphael, 1997).

3. Douglas Hoff, "Repertorizing by Tautopathic Reasoning" [online], http://www.homeoinfo.com/05_repertorizing/tautopathic.php [Nov. 20, 2003].

4. Paracelsus as quoted in Jay Yasgur, *Homeopathic Dictionary* (Greenville, Penn.: Van Hoy Publishers, 1998), p. 71.

5. Another meaning for *constitutional remedy* is a remedy that matches the whole person with a chronic ailment, including physical, mental, and emotional symptoms, as well as personality.

6. Steven Kayne, *Homeopathic Pharmacy* (New York: Churchill Livingston, 1997), p. 155.

7. Jeremy Sherr, *The Dynamics and Methodology of Homeopathic Provings* (Malvern, U.K.: Dynamis Books, 1995), p. 50.

8. Todd Rowe, *Homeopathic Methodology* (Berkeley: North Atlantic Books, 1998), p. 110.

9. Ibid.

10. Steven Olsen, "Letters," *Homeopathy Today* 22, no. 7 (2002): 27.

11. Olsen, "Letters," *Homeopathy Today* 20, no. 11 (2000): 24–25.

12. Karl Robinson, "Symptoms as Arbitrary Phenomena," *Homeopathy Today* 21, no. 12 (2001): 28.

13. Steven Barrett, "Applied Kinesiology: Muscle-Testing for 'Allergies' and 'Nutritional Deficiencies'" [online], http://chirobase.org/06DD/ak.html [Aug. 2, 2002]; Edzard Ernst, editor, *The Desktop Guide to Complementary and Alternative Medicine: An Evidence-Based Approach* (Edinburgh: Mosby, 2001), p. 20.

14. Advertisement, *Homeopathy Today* 21, no. 3 (2001): 17.

15. Even this fundamental principle of classical homeopathy is controversial. According to Ullman, recent research indicates that Hahnemann, in his later years, prescribed two remedies to most of his patients. One remedy was for acute symptoms, the other for the underlying chronic problem. *The Consumer's Guide to Homeopathy* (New York: G.P. Putnam's Sons, 1995), p. 110.

16. Elizabeth Wright-Hubbard, *A Brief Study Course in Homeopathy* (St. Louis: Formur, 1997), pp. 50–51.

17. Bill Gray, Homeopathy: *Science or Myth?* (Berkeley: North Atlantic Books, 2000), p. 123.

18. George Vithoulkas, "A Man with a Mission," Interview with George Vithoulkas, *Homoeopathic Links* 12, no. 4 (1999): 206.

19. Roger Morrison, et al., letter to the editor, *Homeopathy Today* 20, no. 5 (2001): 21.

20. Most historical scientists discussed more concrete concepts than homeopaths did and often expressed concepts in the quantitative language of mathematics; thus there is less doubt about what they meant.

21. Rudi Verspoor and S. Decker, *Homeopathy Re-Examined* (Gloucester, Canada: Hahnemann Center for Heilkunst, 1999).

3. *Remedy Potency*

According to homeopaths, the more dilute a remedy is, the more powerful it is, as long as it has been succussed (or ground and stirred) at each dilution stage. This concept was first proposed by Samuel Hahnemann nearly two centuries ago. Contemporary homeopaths do not question this principle, which is believed to be valid even for dilutions that go way beyond the point at which any of the original medicinal material could remain. Thus, the healing power in homeopathic remedies is nonmolecular. The claim that **nonmolecular remedies** are biologically active contradicts almost all of chemistry, biology, and conventional medicine, wherein molecules are the active ingredients and the fewer molecules, the weaker the effect. Homeopathy offers no proven theories for the active "ingredient" in such remedies, or for how living systems could be affected by such remedies. In this chapter, some of the theories and data related to homeopathy's nonmolecular remedies are critically examined.

REMEDIES DO NOT NEED THEIR MOLECULES

As dilution proceeds in the process of remedy preparation, a point will be reached at which essentially none of the original medicinal molecules is left in one sugar pill or one drop of remedy.[1] By the time a remedy is diluted up to 12C and 24X, the chances of a remaining molecule are negligible. For many remedies, the molecules are gone at much lower dilutions (see appendix 2).

To emphasize this point, consider 30C remedies, a common potency. The odds of getting a single original molecule in a pill of a 30C remedy are so low that a patient would have to consume pills equivalent in mass to nearly one billion times the mass of the Earth to get a single such molecule. For a 30C liquid remedy, one would need to consume an amount whose volume is about ten billion times the volume of the Earth to get a single original molecule.

Here is another way to try to grasp the dilution of a 30C remedy. One drop of juice from a plant is sufficient to make 8×10^{61} 30C pellets—enough doses to give one pellet every day to every person on one planet for every star in every solar system in every galaxy in each of billions of universes from the beginning to the inhabitable end of each universe.[2] The mass of sugar needed to make all the pellets would be more than the estimated mass of the known universe!

Homeopaths have acknowledged for the last one hundred and fifty years that no original medicinal molecules are left in their higher-potency remedies. Even in the lower-potency remedies, the molecules do not seem to contribute to the healing power since remedies with more molecules are considered less potent. There is universal agreement that the original medicinal molecules cannot be an active part of most homeopathic remedies.

DILUTION AND BASIC PHYSICS

Pictured in fig. 3.1 is an antique full bottle of 30C Radium bromide pellets with a thin lead sheet formed around the bottle and the label placed on top of the lead. Presumably the lead is intended to protect the pharmacist, the homeopath, and perhaps the patient from the potentially dangerous ionizing radiation that emanates from radium and its inevitable decay products. The lead wrap doubtless seems like a reasonable precaution, but it is unnecessary for the following reasons:

- This is a 30C remedy. There is less than one chance in about 10^{34}, or one in 10,000,000,000,000,000,000,000,000,000,000,000, of finding a single atom of radium in the entire bottle.
- Much more than a single atom would be needed to constitute a hazard, in part because one atom would have only one chance in two of sending out any radiation in the next 1,600 years (its half life), and in part because it takes on the order of billions of such hits of radiation to result in a 1 percent chance of getting cancer. We are subjected to thousands of hits every second from natural sources, with no measurable adverse effects.

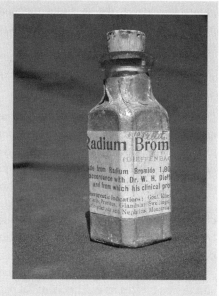

- Radium emits alpha particles that would be completely shielded by the glass bottle alone.
- Some of the decay products of radium emit gamma radiation, which is much more penetrating then alpha particles. The thin layer of lead would offer essentially no protection against such gamma radiation. Lead has no magical shielding ability; it is mass that matters. In this case, the bottle itself does more shielding than the lead because the glass has more mass than the lead wrapping.

HOW CAN REMEDIES WITH NO MEDICINAL MOLECULES WORK?

The claimed action of medicines is easier to accept if there is a logical explanation of how it works. For instance, the shape of a drug molecule might make it fit into a particular protein molecule associated with a disease, interfering with its action; or, if a drug claims to work by preventing a virus from replicating, or by changing the pH of a body fluid, these claims can often be checked in test tube (in vitro) experiments. None of this proves that the medicine will work for people, but it makes its effectiveness more plausible. Proven theories and mechanisms can also lead to the development of improved or additional medicines. Thus it is useful as well as reassuring to find explanations for how remedies work.

Proposed Theories

It is not easy to explain how a medicine works when it has no molecules as active ingredients; below are some theories proposed by Hahnemann and by today's homeopaths. The people who have proposed these theories include practitioners and researchers. The reader is not expected to understand all these theories; neither do I. Some may be metaphors more than specific testable theories.

To begin with, Hahnemann stated, "By means of this mechanical processing . . . a given medicinal substance . . . is subtilized and transformed by these higher and higher dynamizations to become a spirit-like medicinal power."[3]

Miranda Castro suggests an electrochemical pattern: "One theory is that the succussion creates an electrochemical pattern which is stored in the dilutant and which then spreads like liquid crystal through the body's own water. Another hypothesis suggests that the dilution process triggers an electromagnetic imprinting which directly affects the electromagnetic field of the body."[4]

Dr. F. K. Bellokossy espouses electric fields: "We then produce electric fields around every particle of the powdered drug; and the more we triturate (grind), the stronger electric fields we produce, and the more potentized becomes the triturated material."[5]

John Cain favors magnetism: "A slight magnetic code is made that carries forward and amplifies the unique bio-signature of the starting compound."[6]

George Vithoulkas speaks of energy:

> The energy which is contained in a limited form in the original substance is somehow released and transmitted to the molecules of the solvent. Once the original substance is no longer present, the remaining energy in the solvent can be continually enhanced *ad infinitum*. The solvent molecules have taken on the dynamic energy of the original substance. We know from clinical results that the therapeutic energy still retains the "vibrational frequency" of the original substance, but the energy has been enhanced to such a degree that it is capable of stimulating the dynamic plane of the patient sufficiently to produce a cure.[7]

Wayne Jonas and Jennifer Jacobs mention many different mechanisms:

It is now well known that water and water/alcohol mixtures are not simply uniform dispersions of molecules and atoms, but that they often arrange themselves in certain patterns called coherence patterns. There are a number of possible ways these patterns might be stabilized and propagated through subsequent dilutions during the succussion or agitation process. These possible mechanisms include: (1) **clathrate** [boldface added] formation (in which water molecules form "clusters" in specific patterns that mimic the chemicals that they dissolve); (2) isotopic self-organization effects of oxygen isotopes (in which "heavy" water molecules channel specific information because their molecular "spins" are unique from regular water molecules); (3) electrodynamic polarization fields (in which electromagnetic energy such as light organize other molecules with which they come into contact); and (4) coherent excitation (in which molecules vibrating at one frequency will "activate" other molecules in a similar "octave" just as a middle C on the piano will get other "C" notes to vibrate without direct contact).[8]

Several theoretical mechanisms have been proposed to account for such observations, one of which involves the transfer of the "disregulatory" (or unhealthy) electrical field of the patient to the remedy by coupling of "biophotons." Instead of the signal being localized and coming from the medication, the signal comes from the patient, is coupled, absorbed, or dispersed through the remedy, releasing the unhealthy state in the individual.[9]

Some theorists suggest that intentionality and consciousness must be brought to any explanation of how non-local, and nonspecific, quantum potentials might be "collapsed" into so-called informational coherence patterns (molecules), which then have specific effects.[10]

William Pensinger, Douglas Paine, and Julia Jus espouse a rather more complex theory:

> Potentizing homeopathic substances beyond the Avogadro limit is a critical-state coherent process, wherein an element of active information cannot be considered identical to itself. Temporal ordering is paramount in transforming such information to and from the quantal base state, and requires m-valued logics and skew-parallel geometries to represent the identity transparency produced by the active temporal operators. . . . In homeopathic potentization the dilution-succussion process . . . becomes a water-borne stack of crisis states that cascade highly organized (i.e., coherent) time-pattern shapes through the nested collection of "acetate" clock-sheets constituting the transparent information ground."[11]

This last quotation uses some terminology from contemporary physics, but it is not physics as understood by physicists. I have absolutely no idea what this means, and neither do some of my scientist colleagues. Chemist Lionel Milgrom recently reviewed a homeopathy book and made a comment that may well be applicable here: "I have to say I find Lessell's opinions (they are not theories) to be an uncritical procession of mental meanderings randomly garnered from a variety of popular physics and fringe science sources."[12]

HOMEOPATHY IS NOT HERBAL MEDICINE

Some members of the public confuse homeopathy with many other complimentary/alternative approaches to health care, but especially with herbal medicine. The only similarity between homeopathy and herbal medicine is that some of homeopathy's remedies are made starting with herbs. Otherwise, they resemble each other very little.

Homeopathic remedies are taken in tiny amounts (a few drops or a few tiny sugar pills). Herbs are taken in significant amounts, for example a cup of "tea" or a concentrated pill. Many homeopathic remedies are so dilute that none of the original molecules are left, and it makes little difference how much is taken (chapter 6). Herbs are molecular remedies and it matters very much how much is taken; overdosing and underdosing are both possible.

Homeopathic remedies require succussion to gain power. The power in herbal remedies is the herb.

Although some homeopathic remedies are made from herbs, many are not, including remedies based on polystyrene, plutonium, diamond, human body parts and fluids, snake venom, and granite. Homeopaths believe that everything is a potential homeopathic remedy. Herbalists restrict themselves mostly to herbs.

Homeopaths discover what a remedy can cure primarily through provings. Herbalists do not; herbs need not induce symptoms in healthy people in order to be useful remedies. The utility of herbs is, in principle, based only on evidence they cure, just as in conventional medicine.

Homeopathic prescriptions are individualized; two people with the same ailment or disease rarely receive the same remedy because unusual symptoms apparently unrelated to the patient's ailment or disease are critical to selecting the remedy. Herbs are selected primarily on the ailment or disease; hence two patients with the same ailment are likely to be given the same herb.

Scientifically it is plausible that herbs could have medicinal effects because they are molecular remedies, although this is not to say that all or even most claims for herbs have been scientifically proven. At present, there is no plausible explanation for why homeopathy's nonmolecular remedies should have any effect.

Plausibility

Conventional science and engineering are based on the materialist assumption that known physical things, such as molecules, atoms, electrons, protons, neutrons, fields (electric, magnetic, and gravitational), and known types of radiation are the building blocks of the universe. Of course, not all phenomena have been explained, but it appears at this time that no verified phenomenon is inconsistent with this view of the world. None of the homeopathic theories just cited has been needed to explain any incontrovertibly established observations outside of homeopathy. Billions of nonhomeopathic experiments have been conducted in all fields of science throughout the world, all predicated on the materialist view of the world. If the homeopaths are right, many and repeated experiments should have revealed phenomena inexplicable by current science and explainable by one of the homeopathic theories. However, none has been verified beyond reasonable doubt. This does not mean that homeopathic remedies cannot work, but it does mean that the scientific community will ask for very strong evidence to be convinced that they do.

NONCLINICAL EVIDENCE FOR ACTIVITY OF NONMOLECULAR SOLUTIONS

For homeopaths, the most convincing evidence that remedies are effective is that their patients often get better after taking the remedies. We will take a critical look at this evidence in chapter 10.

Another kind of evidence does not involve healing effects on people, but rather laboratory measurements of various types. Results here have no direct bearing on the efficacy of practical homeopathy, but any evidence that solutions diluted beyond the molecular limit are different from pure solvents would be a significant step and would be very startling to, and hence exciting for, the scientific world.

Some published research in this area is favorable[13] and some is unfavorable to the hypothesis that nonmolecular preparations have measurable properties.[14] Most of the research has not been convincingly duplicated by different scientists. Three examples are discussed below.

Nuclear Magnetic Resonance

Nuclear magnetic resonance (NMR), a technique that is sensitive to detailed molecular structure and environments, involves the same fundamental physics as the magnetic resonance imaging (MRI) that is so powerful as a medical diagnostic tool. A number of NMR studies have claimed that homeopathic remedies diluted past the molecular limit show differences compared with pure solvent or equally diluted and succussed solvent that did not start with any medicinal material.[15]

Recently, there have been two replication efforts, and both failed. Aabel et al. attempted to reproduce Weingärtner's results[16] and concluded: "There is no experimental evidence that homeopathic remedies make any kind of imprint on their solvent which can be detected with nuclear magnetic resonance."[17]

Milgrom et al. could not replicate Roland Conte's results,[18] and in this case found the probable error in Conte's work: "We conclude therefore that the differences in T2 earlier observed by Conte et al. using low-resolution NMR, are due to the experimental artifact of silica and impurity leaching from the walls of his (soda-glass) NMR tubes."[19]

Benveniste's Experiment

The best-known work on nonmolecular solutions is the paper by French scientist Jacques Benveniste and his colleagues published in *Nature* in 1988.[20] The authors claimed to have measured biological activity of homeopathically prepared solutions via the human basophil degranulation test, a standard test for investigating allergic sensitivity.

The results were very intriguing. Solutions way past the molecular limit appeared still to be active in this laboratory experiment (this was not a test on humans). Both dilution and succussion were required. This remarkable result seemed to support that nonmolecular homeopathic remedies were active, at least outside of human bodies. However, the experiment contradicted what most homeopaths believe about remedy strength—that it always increases with increasing potency (the number of dilution/succussions). In contrast, the experimenters saw the solutions' activity go up and *down* and up and *down* many times as the potency steadily increased (figure 3.2). Some other experiments have reported similar repetitive up and down variations but with different potencies being most and least active.[21]

Controversy dogged this paper even before it was published. Because the conclusions conflicted so strikingly with known science, it was published along with an explanatory editorial and two rebuttals. After publication, the publisher sent a delegation to Benveniste's lab to observe the pro-

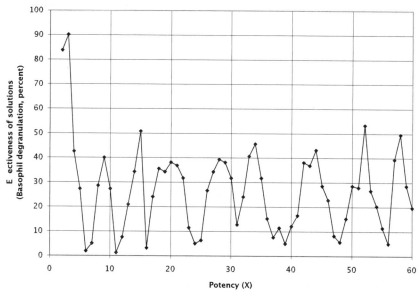

Figure 3.2. Benveniste data. The graph covers potencies from 2X to 60X. Reconstructed from graphed data in E. Davenas et al., "Human Basophil Degranulation Triggered by Very Dilute Antiserum Against IgE," *Nature* 333 (1988): 816–18.

cedures in a replication effort of some of the work. The results were not duplicated, and the delegation concluded,

> The care with which the experiments reported have been carried out did not match the extraordinary character of the claims made in the interpretation. . . . The phenomena described are not reproducible, but there has been no serious investigation of the reason. . . . The data lack errors of the magnitude that would be expected and which are unavoidable. . . . No serious attempt has been made to eliminate systematic errors, including observer bias. . . . The climate of the laboratory is inimical to an objective evaluation of the exceptional data.[22]

The Benveniste affair has become one of the most contentious issues between homeopaths and scientists. Quite a large number of replications have been attempted, with mixed results: Some contradicted the original results,[23] while others have supported the original paper.[24] Emotions are high, and homeopaths tend to interpret the skepticism of scientists as close-mindedness or as some sort of conspiracy.[25]

The fact that at this time there is a mix of positive and negative results is of interest in a historical context. Cold fusion, and other physics mistakes, started out with roughly half the published papers in support, and half finding no effect; it took a while for a scientific consensus to emerge. We now know that cold fusion does not occur as reported in the original paper. The enthusiasm and belief of some of the scientists had resulted in carelessness and unconscious bias in their work.

Conspiracy or not, the Benveniste result is ultimately a scientific issue, and only science can resolve it. Because of the extraordinary nature of the claim, the scientific community reasonably requires extraordinary proof; such proof involves many replications with consistently strong positive results conducted by many different reputable researchers using the best methodology. This threshold has not been reached.

Memory of Water

An often-mentioned theory is that water has "memory" of what was dissolved in it. A commonly cited mechanism is **water clusters** or *clathrates*. These water molecule clusters reportedly form around some of the original medicinal molecules, forming structures that are unique to each homeopathic remedy. The idea of self-replicating structures seems to have been first proposed by G. S. Anagnostatos.[26] The clusters can also replicate themselves in the absence of the original molecules, as is needed to explain further increases in potency after all the original medicinal molecules are lost to dilution. Succussion is thought to help the water molecules arrange themselves into the clusters.

There was considerable excitement in the homeopathic community starting around 1996 when Dr. Shui-Yin Lo of American Technologies Group reported verifying the existence of such clusters in liquid water.[27] He termed them "IE" crystals—for ice formed under the influence of electric fields—but they appear to be the same as the hypothesized water clusters or clathrates. He claimed both a theoretical basis for IE crystals and electrical and spectroscopic measurements verifying their existence.

The existence of *stable* clusters of water molecules at room temperature would be remarkable. Dr. Lo's company makes extraordinary claims for IE clusters. They are the active ingredient in plastic balls containing blue liquid that supposedly replace detergents and last for many, many loads of laundry; they are also the active ingredient in "the Force," a device which when placed in an automobile's air filter dramatically improves gas mileage according to the claims. The Oregon Department of

Justice has declared both products to be ineffective and to be based on false claims.[28] Independent scientists have pointed out that Lo's claims violate the laws of thermodynamics.[29]

If water clusters exist, many observable effects should distinguish them from pure plain water, and the magnitude of these effects should change with potency as the concentration of clusters in the water increases. The measurable properties should include density, compressibility, viscosity, electrical conductivity, thermal conductivity, refractive index, osmotic pressure, specific and latent heat, and dielectric properties. Some research has reported such evidence, specifically on dielectric and thermal properties,[30] and the nuclear magnetic resonance evidence reported above, but the results have not yet met the high standards required given the unusual nature of the claims.

The water cluster explanation of **water memory** also contradicts many claims in homeopathy, such as limitless potentizability (the number of available water molecules is finite), the existence of imponderable remedies (around what do the clusters form?), the effectiveness of dry forms not involving water molecules such as sugar pellets and triturated remedies, and more (see appendix 3). We appear to be a long way from a satisfactory theory for nonmolecular remedies.

THOUGHTS ON SUCCUSSION

Hahnemann's instructions for succussion are, "Give the tightly corded vial 100 strong succussions with the hand against a hard but elastic body (such as a leather-bound book)."[31] Some pharmacists go to great lengths to faithfully replicate this process, even in automated manufacturing. Swirling, stirring, or shaking is not considered adequate by some homeopaths.

Homeopaths do not agree on how much succussion is appropriate. Recommendations typically range from twenty to one hundred shakes or poundings, and from ten seconds to two and one-half minutes,[32] but some homeopaths use just a few shakes.

Why must remedies be agitated at all beyond what is needed to mix the ingredients? Why must remedies be agitated in this particular way? Why would succussing have a different impact than swirling or stirring? Are the turbulence, shear, air incorporation, and acceleration significantly different in succussion? Since homeopathy has no plausible scientific theory for the active ingredient in remedies, there can be as yet no plausible theory why remedies must be shaken, not stirred. Apparently it is done primarily because Hahnemann so instructed.

Some homeopaths ignore Hahnemann's leather book instructions, believing other methods of mixing/shaking are effective:

- Historically and even today, some remedy preparation methods do not involve much succussion (as defined by Hahnemann). For instance, the **fluxion method** of remedy preparation involves continuous dilution (with some intentional turbulence due to flowing water) until the desired dilution is reached, followed by just a few succussions. Many homeopaths who have used such remedies find that they work just as well as remedies succussed at every stage of dilution.[33] LM remedies also involve much less succussion for the same dilutions than do the more common centesimal remedies.
- Hahnemann warned against carrying liquid remedies on one's body[34]—the jostling could increase the potencies to dangerous levels, even though such jostling is not the same as pounding the remedy bottles on a leather-bound book.
- Sometimes homeopaths recommend that a liquid remedy bottle be shaken a few times before taking it to raise its potency.
- Many homeopaths believe that they can further potentize pill or liquid remedies by diluting them in a glass of water and stirring with a spoon, not pounding a closed container against a leather-bound book. R. U. Ramakrishnan says that stirring alone, without dilution, increases the potency of his homeopathic cancer remedies.[35]
- Last but not least, triturated remedies are not succussed at all and yet are treated as having the same potency as those that are.

So, do the details of succussion matter? Does succession itself matter? The normal scientific approach to resolving such issues is simply to test remedies for their strengths. However, homeopathy has no laboratory test for its remedies and consequently must rely on indirect evidence, such as the effects on patients. In clinical trials, potency has hardly been addressed, much less the details of succussion; it has proven sufficiently challenging just to show that a remedy improves health, without regard to such details as potency. Thus, we reach the end of the line—the importance of and techniques for succussion cannot be determined with any certainty at this time. They remain a mystery.

WHY *DILUTE* PAST 12C AND 24X?

Past 12C and 24X, there are essentially no original medicinal molecules left. Why would continued dilution matter? All that is claimed to be present is the "memory," "information," "energy," or "vibration" of the original molecules, perhaps in the form of water molecule clusters, which can ostensibly generate more of the same on succussion. Then why not just do extra succussions of a 12C remedy rather than bothering with the dilutions? Each dilution can only decrease the amount of the "energy" since 99 percent of the potentized liquid is discarded at each C stage. Dilution makes some sense for reducing side effects when the concentration of the original material is high; but once past that problem, dilution seems only wasteful. A likely reason why homeopaths continue to dilute past 12C is that Hahnemann did not realize that no original medicinal molecules were left at this dilution, and homeopaths are inclined to faithfully reproduce what he did regardless of new information.

CONCLUSION

The claim that medicinal power increases as the dilution increases is probably the single most difficult point for skeptics to accept and for homeopathy to defend. It runs counter to common sense and to scientific knowledge of the world.

It is remarkable enough that nature has provided us with millions of different materials and compounds—through the intricacies of how atoms bond to each other. Homeopathy would have us believe there is an entire mirror world of homeopathic remedies (a distinct remedy for every material and compound) with the same variety and complexity and number of entities, each of which has a powerful and unique health effect. It is not surprising that many people ask for substantial evidence before accepting this claim.

Whatever active agent is proposed for homeopathic remedies, homeopathy would be more credible if the agent were measurable. The amount of this agent should increase with increasing dilution and succussion. The mechanism by which this agent interacts with the human body to stimulate healing should have convincing experimental (and theoretical) support. Researchers Harald Walach and Wayne Jonas summarize the physical and biological research as follows:

The most frequent observation is that there are often interesting initial results, highly significant, seemingly clear cut. . . . But when probed for stable, independent replicability, not one has so far been proved so robust that the effects would be reproducible even by a believer, let alone a skeptic. . . . None so far can cover all phenomena or is empirically tested well enough to support any of the bold claims put forward by homeopathic enthusiasts.[36]

In the current absence of convincing direct laboratory evidence for an active ingredient and its mode of action, homeopathy must rely primarily on indirect and more problematic evidence—the effects on patients (see chapter 11).

When Hahnemann was developing homeopathy, he could not have known that no medicinal molecules were left in the higher potency remedies he used. Although there was good evidence for the atomic nature of matter, there was no quantitative estimate of atomic size until after Hahnemann's death. Hahnemann died in 1843, and the first calculation of the value of Avogadro's number (which is related to the size of atoms) was performed around 1865. After Hahnemann's death, when it became clear that many homeopathic potencies contained no original medicinal molecules, homeopaths had three choices—abandon super-dilute remedies as impossible, continue believing in Hahnemann's metaphysical explanations of the remedies' potency, or try to find a scientific explanation for how they could work. All three paths have been taken.

NOTES

1. The *original medicinal molecules* are the molecules from the salt, belladonna, Arnica, or whatever was used at the start of the process.

2. I have generously assumed 100 billion people per planet, one inhabitable planet per star, 10^{23} stars in the known universe, and the life-friendly duration of a universe to be 100 billion years. The results are not very sensitive to these assumptions.

3. Samuel Hahnemann, Aphorism 270, *Organon of the Medical Art*, 6th ed., edited and annotated by Wenda O'Reilly (Redmond, Wash.: Birdcage Books, 1996).

4. Miranda Castro, *The Complete Book of Homeopathy* (New York: St. Martin's Press, 1990), pp. 12–13.

5. Quoted by Maesimuns B. Panos and Jane Heimlich, "What Is Homeopathy?" [online], http://www.jacktips.com/homeopathy.htm [Nov. 29, 2002].

6. John W. Cain, "What Is Homeopathy and How Is a Homeopathic Product Made?" [online], http://www.celletech.com/info/homomade.htm [Nov. 29, 2002].

7. George Vithoulkas, *The Science of Homeopathy* (New York: Grove Press, 1980), p. 104.

8. Wayne Jonas and Jennifer Jacobs, *Healing with Homeopathy: The Doctors' Guide* (New York: Warner Books, 1996), p. 87.

9. Ibid., p. 89.

10. Ibid., pp. 90–91.

11. William L. Pensinger, Douglas A. Paine, and Julia Jus, "Time-Logics of the Quantal Base State in Homeopathic Potentization," *Journal of the American Institute of Homeopathy* 90, no. 2 (1997): 77–88.

12. Lionel Milgrom, book review of Colin Lessell's *A New Physics of Homeopathy, Homeopathy* 92, no. 1 (2003): 61.

13. See, for example, Jurgen Schulte and P. Christian Endler, editors, *Ultra High Dilution: Physics and Physiology* (Dordrecht, Netherlands: Kluwer Academic Publishers, 1994).

14. See, for example, P. Fisher et al., "The Influence of the Homeopathic Remedy Plumbum Metallicum on the Excretion Kinetics of Lead in Rats," *Human Toxicology* 6 (1987): 321–24.

15. T. M. Young, "Nuclear Magnetic Resonance Studies of Succussed Solutions: A Preliminary Report," *Journal of the American Institute of Homeopathy* 68 (1975): 8–16.; A. D. Sacks, "Nuclear Magnetic Resonance Spectroscopy of Homeopathic Remedies," *Journal of Holistic Medicine* 5 (1983): 172–77; O. Weingärtner, "NMR-Features That Relate to Homeopathic Sulphur-Potencies," *Berlin Journal of Research in Homeopathy* 1 (1990): 61–68; J. L. Demangeat and C. Demangeat, "Modifications des temps de relaxation RMN à 4 Mhz des protons du solvant dans les très hautes dilutions salines de silice/lactose," *Journal of Medical and Nuclear Biophysics* 2 (1992): 135–45; R. R. Conte et al., *Theory of High Dilutions and Experimental Aspects* (Paris: Polytechnica, 1996).

16. Weingärtner.

17. S. Aabel, S. Fossheim, and F. Rise, "Nuclear Magnetic Resonance (NMR) Studies of Homeopathic Solutions," *British Homeopathic Journal* 90 (2001):14–20.

18. Conte et al.

19. L. R. Milgrom et al., "On the Investigation of Homeopathic Potencies Using Low Resolution NMR T2 Relaxation Times: An Experimental and Critical Survey of the Work of Roland Conte et al.," *British Homeopathic Journal* 90 (2001): 5–13.

20. E. Davenas et al., "Human Basophil Degranulation Triggered by Very Dilute Antiserum Against IgE," *Nature* 333 (1988): 816–18.

21. For a summary with references of such research, see James Stephenson, "A Review of Investigations into the Action of Substances in Solutions Greater than 1×10^{-24} (Microdilutions)," *Journal of the American Institute of Homeopathy* 48, no. 11 (1995): 79–94.

22. J. Maddox, J. Randi, and W. Stewart, "'High-Dilution' Experiments a Delusion," *Nature* 334 (1988): 287–90.

23. S. J. Hirst et al., "Human Basophil Degranulation Is Not Triggered by Very Dilute Antiserum Against Human IgE," *Nature* 366 (1993): 525–27; J. Seagrave, "Evidence of Non-reproducibility," *Nature* 334 (1998): 559; and S. Bonini, E. Adriani, and F. Balsano, "Evidence of Non-reproducibility," *Nature* 334 (1988): 559.

24. P. Belon et al., "Inhibition of Human Basophil Degranulation by Successive Histamine Dilutions: Results of a European Multi-centre Trial," *Inflammation Research* 48, Supplement 1 (1999): S17–S18.

25. See, for instance, Michel Schiff, *The Memory of Water* (San Francisco: Thorsons, 1995).

26. G. S. Anagnostatos, "Small Water Clusters (Clathrates) in the Homeopathic Preparation Process," in *Ultra High Dilution: Physics and Physiology*, ed. P. Christian Endler and Jurgen Schulte (Dordrecht, Netherlands: Kluwer Academic Publishers, 1994), pp. 121–28.

27. Shui-Yin Lo, "Anomalous State of Ice," *Modern Physics Letters B* 10, no. 19 (1996): 909–19; Shui-Yin Lo et al., "Physical Properties of Water with I_E Structures," *Modern Physics Letters B* 10, no. 19 (1996): 921–30.

28. D. Touretzky, "ATG Investigation: The Oregon Files" [online], http://www2.cs.cmu.edu/~dst/ATG/oregon.html [Aug. 3, 2002].

29. Paul Engelking, e-mail [online], http://www.cs.cmu.edu/~dst/ATG/engelking/engelking-analysis.txt [Aug. 3, 2002].

30. For a summary, see Gerassimos S. Anagnostatos et al, "Theory and Experiments on High Dilutions," in *Homeopathy: A Critical Appraisal*, ed. Edzard Ernst and Eckhart G. Hahn (Woburn, Mass.: Butterworth-Heinemann, 1998), pp. 153–66.

31. Hahnemann, Aphorism 270. The number of succussions in this quotation refers to LM remedies.

32. Steven Kayne, *Homeopathic Pharmacy* (New York: Churchill Livingston, 1997), p. 49.

33. According to Julian Winston, "There are many homeopaths still using fluxion potencies from their stock, and they seem to work very well." Lyghtforce e-mail list, *Homeopathy Digest* 2, no. 220 (2001), archives at http://www.lyghtforce.com/HomeoList/ [online].

34. Anthony Campbell, *Homeopathy in Perspective*, chapter 3, [online], http://www.accampbell.uklinux.net/homeopathy/index.html [March 11, 2002].

35. R. U. Ramakrishnan and Catherine R. Coulter, *A Homeopathic Approach to Cancer* (St. Louis: Quality Medical Publishing, 2001), p. 3.

36. Harald Walach and Wayne B. Jonas, "Homeopathy," in *Clinical Research in Complementary Therapies*, ed. George Lewith, Wayne B. Jonas, and Harald Walach (London: Churchill Livingstone, 2002), pp. 233, 234.

4. *Provings*

This chapter takes a closer look at provings. The primary objective is to assess the claim that the observed symptoms are caused by the remedies. Most provings fall far short of modern scientific methodological standards, the weakest link being the absence of a standard control group and corresponding statistical analysis. Many of the detailed procedures encourage **false positives**—symptoms not caused by the remedy. A detailed look at the symptoms themselves casts doubt on their claimed cause. Interestingly, homeopaths do not always value more data; too many data are believed to cloud rather than clarify the differences among remedies. The most telling fact is that the provings with the best methodological quality yield very few if any symptoms attributable to the remedy.

This is a long chapter. Readers more interested in other topics are invited to skip to the summary and conclusions at the end of this chapter.

INTERNAL AND EXTERNAL REALITY

The contrasting concepts of internal and external reality are essential for understanding some of the material introduced in this chapter and much of the rest of this book.

In most cases when a witness testifies about a crime scene, or when an adult recalls a childhood event, the witness honestly conveys his or her memory. Nonetheless, a memory is not necessarily an accurate recording of events. The memory and the physical event are both real, but their contents need not coincide. Memory is very susceptible to change over time and can even be created by suggestion alone.[1] Memory is part of a person's **internal reality**; what actually happened is part of **external reality**. In general, memories, perceptions, beliefs, and feelings are a person's internal reality, whereas the physical world, as verified using the methods of science, is external reality.

For example, two centuries ago, many physicians believed that draining blood from a sick person would help the patient heal. This belief was real; it was an internal reality. However, the external reality is that draining blood is usually detrimental to health. As another example, astrologers are convinced that positions of heavenly bodies influence people's lives; they perceive astrology being verified every day; it feels real. However, scientific tests fail to correlate the positions of heavenly bodies with people's personalities or events in their lives. Astrology is an internal reality for those who believe in it but appears to have no external reality.

Internal reality—what we feel, perceive, think, and believe—is in a sense all that directly matters to people. What more is there for us as individuals? In no way should we belittle its existence or value. But external reality—the physical world that can be measured—is also important. We live in this world and are dependent on it for our existence and survival.

External reality can never be known with absolute certainty; our interpretation of it is always subject to refutation. When supportive evidence accumulates, confidence increases, and pragmatic certainty can emerge: Few would doubt that if they stepped off a roof, they would accelerate downward. Nonetheless, our knowledge of external reality is always subject to revision. In contrast, internal reality is always certain; whatever we perceive and feel is what we perceive and feel even if ambiguous or unclear.

Internal reality is subjective and individual. We do not perceive or remember events exactly the same way as anyone else, and we do not have identical feelings about them. External reality is objective; the goal of science is to describe nature itself. If Einstein had not been born, someone else would have come up with the theory of relativity. Different words might have been coined, and different symbols used in the equations, but since relativity is simply a description of nature, the basic concepts and mathematics would have been equivalent no matter who first wrote them down. (This is not the case in the arts. Had Brahms not composed his first symphony, no one else would have done so. Artists' contributions to culture are unique, whereas scientists' are not.) Science strives for a description of nature that is independent of our internal individuality. External reality does not depend on personal experiences, personal training, personal preference, cultural comfort, personal belief, or on personal interpretation of external conditions. Believing that one would hover after stepping off a roof has no impact on what actually happens.

Homeopaths maintain that their remedies are responsible for prover responses; that is the homeopaths' internal reality. The focus of this chapter is the exploration of the external reality of this causal relation.

SHOULD PROVINGS PRODUCE SYMPTOMS?

For the purpose of discussing provings, it is useful to classify homeopathic remedies into four categories: *toxic*, *infectious*, *harmless*, and *empty* (see table 4.1).

Table 4.1. Toxicity-Based Classification for Source Material in Homeopathic Remedies		
Category	**Comment**	**Examples**
Toxic	Harmful in small doses	Arsenic, belladonna, mercury, plutonium
Infectious	Derived directly from disease agents or infected tissue and hence originally containing pathogens	Blood from AIDS patient, dog excrement, parasites, yeast
Harmless[a]	Harmless due to relative chemical inertness or because it is a food	Milk, neon, water, whole wheat bread, chocolate
Empty	Not material (imponderables)— undetectable in tincture even before any dilution	Green light, x-rays, magnetic fields, wind, moonlight

a. Harmless to most people; some individuals may be allergic.

This classification scheme is primarily conceptual. There is a continuum between toxic and harmless materials. The dose matters. All materials in sufficiently large quantities can be harmful, and no material in sufficiently small quantities is harmful. For instance, salt is not usually considered toxic, yet three-quarters of a cup ingested all at once can be fatal. Similarly, a 10 **g** dose of caffeine taken at once can be fatal, but a daily cup of coffee which on the average contains 0.1 g of caffeine, is not.

Ordinary chemical effects are impossible at or above a potency of about 24X or 12C because essentially none of the original molecules is left. Chemical effects are extremely unlikely even above just 10X or 5C because the dilution is ten billion or higher, and few toxic materials have measurable effects when so dilute. The distribution of dilutions used in all provings published in the United Kingdom between 1945 and 1995 indicates a wide range of potencies, from 1X to 200C.[2] The most common potencies in these provings were 6C, 12C, and 30C. None of these potencies is likely to have any biochemical effect. Infectious materials are sterilized and are also diluted so much (typically to 30C or higher) that there are no pathogens left in the remedy. Remedies based on food should cause no symptoms aside from a possible allergic reaction from very low-potency remedies. Chemically inert materials should produce no symptoms at any dilution. **Imponderable remedies** can have no chemical effect since they are "empty," to begin with, even without dilution.

Thus, there is no explanation in Western science for why any symptoms would be caused by the remedies administered in most provings. And yet the participants feel a plethora of symptoms in provings.

Much of the following discussion is based on the description of provings by Jeremy Sherr in *The Dynamics and Methodology of Homeopathic Provings*. Sherr is an internationally recognized homeopathy teacher and an expert on provings.

CAUSES OF PROVINGS SYMPTOMS

A typical proving might have twenty subjects. Even though they all may have appeared to be healthy at the beginning of the process, it is likely that some will naturally develop illnesses and assorted symptoms during the few months of the proving. It is essential to identify any symptoms actually caused by the homeopathic remedy, despite scientific improbability, from those that would have occurred anyway. With the help of their supervisors, the provers are asked to classify their own symptoms into the categories indicated in table 4.2. All but the "normal" and "natural" symptoms are then attributed to the remedy.

Table 4.2. Symptom Classification for Remedy Provings	
Symptoms Assumed to Have Been Caused by the Remedy	
New	Symptom never experienced before
Old	Recurrence of earlier symptom not experienced for more than a year
Altered	Change in current or old symptom
Unusual	Unusual symptom for the prover
Cured	Symptom that disappeared during a proving
Under the influence	All symptoms of a prover are to be included if the prover is "under the influence of the remedy"
Symptoms Assumed Not to Have Been Caused by the Remedy	
Normal (also called "*recent*")	Symptom experienced in the last year (before the proving)
Natural	Symptom with known cause other than the homeopathic dose

These categories are loosely defined, and therein lies an almost insurmountable weakness from a scientific point of view. How much alteration is needed to classify a symptom as altered? How unusual to be unusual? How does a prover (or practitioner) know whether a headache is due to the remedy or to a stressful day at work? Is elbow pain remedy-related or due to overuse? Does a cold occur because the remedy increased the prover's susceptibility or simply because of exposure to a virus? The prover cannot know for sure; these decisions are subjective and consequently subject to bias. Moreover, why is the cutoff between "old" and "normal" symptoms one year rather than six months or two years? What is the evidence that this amount of time accurately delineates between symptoms caused and not caused by the remedy?

If a prover has a recurrent or chronic symptom that becomes less intense or disappears during a proving, it is assumed that the remedy cured the symptom. But health can improve for many reasons other than participating in a proving.

Sherr gives some additional guidelines for deciding whether a symptom was caused by the remedy: "The next factor is the perceived meaning of the totality. Once an understanding of the nature of the remedy emerges it may serve to verify or exclude questionable symptoms."[3] This perception will steer a **remedy picture** in a direction that the supervisors believe is appropriate, rather than letting the data speak for themselves. This is not an objective process. Sherr continues, "The inner knowledge and conviction of a prover that these symptoms do not belong to her are a definite and reliable consideration."[4] Here, Sherr is promoting internal reality as external reality, an approach likely to muddy our understanding of external reality. He advises the prover, "If in serious doubt, leave it out."[5] That is good advice, but again the filter is subjective. Once the "nature of the remedy" starts becoming clear, serious doubt may inappropriately disappear.

In addition, most provings are conducted by believers in homeopathy, often students and their teachers at homeopathy schools or attendees at homeopathic meetings or seminars. Thus, the prover may desire to please the organizers or hold other expectations that unconsciously influence the results.

This process of selecting symptoms caused by the remedy appears methodologically weak. How provings should be conducted will be discussed later in this chapter; for now, let us look at the results of provings as typically conducted.

Symptoms Attributed to Remedies

Some of the "symptoms" reported in provings are commonly experienced by healthy people; it is hard to imagine how they could be classified as new, old, altered, or unusual. Hahnemann reported symptoms from oleander including thirst for cold drinks, especially fresh water; great hunger; no appetite; rumbling in the abdomen; weakness of the body; tiredness; laziness: voluptuous dreams; and difficulty sleeping at night.[6] Some recent provings seem to yield almost exclusively symptoms experienced by normal, healthy people, such as desiring alcohol, desiring cold water, desiring sweets, being weary in the afternoon, and having dreams about scary things.[7] Thus, for at least some provers, feeling tired in the afternoon or desiring cold water or sweets must be one of the following:

New: Never experienced before
Old: Not experienced for more than a year before the proving
Altered: A change in a current or old symptom
Unusual: An unusual symptom for the prover

This conclusion seems highly improbable. An alternative explanation for the listing of these common symptoms is that the bar has not been set sufficiently high; the symptom-filtering process is letting in ordinary symptoms that were not caused by the remedy. The question here is not whether the symptoms are real, but whether they are caused by the remedy.

Patients' and Provers' Descriptions

Homeopathy depends on the descriptions of symptoms by patients, as well as provers, specifically in their own particular words.

According to homeopathy, the strength of this approach is that it facilitates a more perfect match between the symptoms of the patient and those of the remedy. The weakness of this approach is that different words may be used to describe the same basic symptoms; if provers and patients happen to use different words for the same symptoms, then the homeopath may overlook the right remedy. One need only look in standard repertories to grasp the problem. All the colors of sputum in Kent's repertory are listed in table 4.3. For each color, a different set of remedies is listed. Thus, it is vital for the patient to judge the color of his sputum accurately, and just as important for the provers to report their colors accurately. But what is the difference between *blue* and *bluish*? Do all provers and patients know the difference among *brownish, bloody brown, brick dust, brownish yellow, dirty looking, liver-colored, muddy-like, prune juice,* and *rusty*? If not, the wrong remedy may be prescribed.

Table 4.3. Sputum Colors, from Kent's Repertory

General Color	Kent's Terms	General Color	Kent's Terms
Black	Blackish	Clear	Glairy
	Dark		Pale
	Blackish yellow		Saliva-like
	Bloody, black		Transparent
	Bloody, dark		Albuminous
		Gray	Ash-colored
Blue	Blue		Dust, as if mixed with
	Bluish		Grayish
			Slate-colored
Brown	Bloody, brown		
	Brick dust	White	White
	Brownish		Calcareous
	Brownish yellow		Cream-like
	Dirty looking		Milky
	Liver-colored		
	Muddy-like		
	Prune juice	Yellow	Lemon-colored
	Rusty		Orange-colored
	Skin, like dead		Purulent
			Yellow
Green	Greenish		

Source: James Tyler Kent, *Repertory of the Homeopathic Materia Medica* (1897–1899; reprint, New Delhi: B. Jain Publishers, 1998), pp. 812–21.

The same questions arise when examining the different textures of sputum listed in Kent's *Repertory* (table 4.4). Will everyone agree on the differences among *globular, granular, lumpy, in masses, in pieces*, and *in the shape of balls*?

Table 4.4. Sputum Textures, from Kent's **Repertory**

Author's Category	Kent's Terms	Author's Category	Kent's Terms
Lumpy	Feels like a round ball	*Ropy*	Membranous
	In shape of balls		Ropey [*sic*]
	Globular	*Thin*	Oleaginous
	Granular		Thin
	Lump, like core of boil		Watery
	Lumpy	*Other*	Breaks and flies like thin batter
	Lumpy, smoke-colored lumps streaked with blood		Bilious
			Cheese, like
	Masses, in		Crumbly
	Pieces, in		Flakes
Hard	Hard		Frothy
	Pasty		Frothy containing blood and mucus
	Thick		
	Tough		Scanty
Slimy	Gelatinous		
	Mucous [adj.]		
	Mucous, bloody		
	Syrup-like		
	Viscid		

Source: James Tyler Kent, *Repertory*, pp. 812–21.

It seems improbable that an exact match between provers' and patients' words is likely to mean much for several reasons: (1) More than one word or phrase is descriptive, and the choice may just be an accident of the words that happened to come to the prover or patient; (2) Since people with many different native languages have conducted provings, we are often looking at translations of the provers' words; translation cannot be an exact process because different languages often do not have words with exactly the same meanings; (3) since the earliest provings were done over two hundred years ago, the meanings of words may have changed over time; and (4) words also have regional, socioeconomic, and ethnic contexts; thus, it is questionable that particular words have absolute meaning.

Extraordinary Time Specificity

In homeopathy, the time of day that symptoms occur is thought to be important. In Kent's repertory, forty-six different quantitative times or time intervals are given for head pain, and each time or time interval has a different list of remedies. The following are a few of the forty-six specific times[8] and their associated remedies that are listed for head pain.

5 A.M.	Calc., kali-bi., kali-i., stann.
6 A.M. until evening	Crot-t.
6 A.M. until 10 A.M.	Arn., lachn., mag-c.
6 A.M. until 3 P.M.	Aur.
6 A.M. until 5 P.M.	Mang.
6 A.M. until 10 P.M.	Phys.
8 A.M.	Bov.
10 A.M.	Apis, ars., bor., cimic., gels., nat-m., thuj.
10 A.M. to 2 P.M.	Alum.
10 A.M. to 3 P.M.	Nat-m.
10 A.M. to 4 P.M.	Stann.
10 A.M. to 6 P.M.	Apis
11 A.M.	Ip., spig., sol-n., sulph.
Noon	Aeth., agar., alum., nat-c., arg-m., arg-n., asar., bell., bov., calc-ar., calc-p., cann-i., carb-v., cedr., cham., chel., chin-s., cic., cob., graph., gymn., ign., indg., jab., kali-bi., kali-n., kalm., lyc., lycps., lyss., mag-c., mang., merc., mur-ac., naja, nat-c., nat-m., phos., puls., rhus-t., spong., sulph., zinc., zing.
1 P.M.	Ail., coca., lyc., mag-c., phys., pic-ac., ptel . . .
2 P.M.	Ars., chel., grat., laur., lyss., phys., ptel. . . .
3 P.M.	Apis, bell., fago., fl-ac., guaj., hura, iber., lycps., lyss., nat-a., sep., sil., thuj., verat-v.
1 A.M.	Pall.

2 A.M.	Cimic., sulph.
3 A.M.	Agar., bov., chin-s., nat-m. thuj.
4 A.M.	Chel., raph., stram.
5 A.M.	Dios., kali-i.[9]

Such a list raises some questions. Why would the remedies Alum., Nat-m., Stann., and Apis. all induce headaches starting at 10 A.M. but lasting four, five, six, and eight hours respectively? Is it plausible that Agar., Bov., Chin-s., Nat-m., and Thuj. all cause headaches at 3 A.M. but not at 2 A.M. or 4 A.M.? Would not headache onset and duration depend on the prover's or patient's recent rest, stress, exercise, and diet? It is hard to believe that the remedies alone control headache timing with the implied precision.

Another interesting feature is that many more remedies are listed at noon than at any other specific time (figure 4.1). The homeopathic interpretation is that many more remedies caused headaches to occur in the provers at noon than at any other specific time. An alternative explanation is that the noon peak is just a reporting artifact due to mental rounding; when a prover said "noon," he or she might have meant "midday"—perhaps any time from 10 A.M. to 2 P.M.

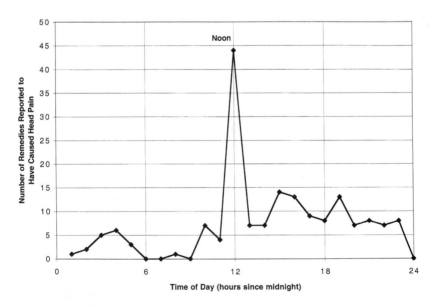

Figure 4.1. Time of day for head pain reported in provings.

Another question comes to mind. When were the remedies taken by the provers? This information is not usually given in repertories or materia medicae. If a remedy tends to induce a headache, one might expect a characteristic delay before its onset, depending on the remedy. Apparently homeopaths see no connection between these times. In their view, some remedies, no matter when taken, induce headaches at very particular times of day.

If these specific times are to be taken seriously, one wonders whether daylight savings time matters. In addition, where one lives within a given time zone can make a difference of as much as an hour in terms of sunrise and sunset and latitude can make much more difference.

The precision implied in the temporal aspects of these data seems questionable. One might wonder whether they represent objective reproducible cause-and-effect reality or merely approximate records of random natural occurrences of ill health.

Opposite Symptoms

An interesting facet of homeopathy is that the same remedy can induce both a particular symptom and its exact opposite. Thus, the same remedy may be called for to cure opposite symptoms (table 4.5).

Table 4.5. Opposite Symptoms from Boericke's Materia Medica

Remedy	Symptoms	
Abrotanum	Diarrhea	Constipation
Natrum muriaticum	Nose: Discharge thin and watery	Nose: Dryness
" "	Fever: Chill between 9 and 11 A.M.	Fever: Heat
Alumina	Stomach: Abnormal cravings	Stomach: No desire to eat
Silicea	Mind: Yielding	Mind: Obstinate
Sulphur	Busy all the time	Loafs—too lazy to rouse himself
"	Complete loss of appetite	Excessive appetite
Veratrum album	Diarrhea	Constipation

Source: Adapted from William Boericke, Materia Medica, 9th ed. (Santa Rosa, Calif.: Boericke and Tafel, 1927).

The experts offer explanations for these opposites. Vithoulkas says,

When a substance is administered to an organism, there are two phases of response. . . . The symptoms generated in this secondary phase can be opposite to those in the primary phase. In any proving, it is important to record symptoms from both phases, even though they appear to be contradictory. Each phase represents a characteristic manifestation of the action of the defense mechanism and therefore must be accorded equal importance.[10]

Sherr finds that the opposite symptoms may appear in either order and argues that **primary and secondary symptoms** should be treated equally.[11]

That a remedy can induce or cure opposite symptoms is so remarkable that one is inclined to consider other explanations. Over the months of a proving, it would not be surprising for some provers to experience opposite symptoms naturally: feeling energetic and tired, having diarrhea and constipation, feeling happy and sad, having a dry and a runny nose. No remedy is required to produce these symptoms. Perhaps this focus of homeopaths on primary and secondary phases of response is a plausible-sounding but unnecessary explanation of opposite symptoms that in fact arise naturally. This would also explain why the order of the symptoms sometimes varies.

Asymmetries

A number of symptoms in repertories and materia medicae are asymmetric, affecting only the left or right portion of the body (table 4.6). Some remedies produce so many one-sided symptoms that they are thought of as one-sided remedies.[12] Some snake venom remedies are in this category.

Table 4.6. Asymmetric Symptoms	
Remedy	**Symptom**
Absinthium	Darting pain in *right* ovary
Radium bromide	*Right* breast soreness
Lac caninum (dog's milk)	Sciatica, *right* side
Natrum muriaticum	Better lying on *right* side
Acetic acid	Aching in *left* jaw
Apis melifica	Swelling in *right* groin

Source: Adapted from Boericke, *Materia Medica*, 9th ed.

There is no doubt that such asymmetric symptoms can occur; we've all had them. The question is whether the cause in a proving is the remedy or something else. Where an organ, such as the heart, is located asymmetrically in the body, asymmetric symptoms are of course possible. However, most of the asymmetric symptoms reported in materia medicae affect body parts that are on average inherently symmetric, such as breasts and jaws. Western science offers no plausible reason why a particular material should consistently produce asymmetric symptoms in healthy people. There are no Western science medications that work for one side of the body but not the other, and there is no known innate asymmetry in body chemistry.

Given the implausibility of asymmetric symptoms in provings, it is reasonable to consider other explanations, for this apparent phenomenon. It is conceivable that they result from previous injuries, asymmetric body build, and asymmetric life habits (e.g., standing, sitting, walking, sleeping, and handedness).

Symptoms Do Not Come Easily

As previously indicated, the symptoms themselves suggest that the remedy may not always be causative. When we examine some of the guidelines for provings, it appears probable that the process elevates ordinary symptoms to remedy-caused status and that some symptoms may only be imagined.

Sherr, for example, states:

> It was evident in the early 1980's that not many provings were being undertaken, and the provings that I did know of had yielded few symptoms. I found it strange that these provings did not produce results and upon further investigation, I came to the conclusion that in most cases this was due to methodology. In retrospect it appeared that symptoms were produced but that due to poor supervision these had passed unnoticed. . . . Therefore meticulous supervision and scrupulous extraction of information are the main principles that I have adopted in my provings. This is the guarantee of accurate and reliable results.[13]

He continues:

> Often when a prover is proving a remedy they don't actually realize that they are experiencing a proving, unless the symptoms are very physical, external or blatant. The prover becomes the proving and therefore they cannot actually perceive that they are changing. . . .

On the third day of the Hydrogen proving I held a meeting of supervisors and provers to discuss the developments so far. Quite a few reported that nothing had happened. As this seemed impossible . . . , I explained that provers would often not notice anything was happening. I sent the supervisors back to investigate the provers thoroughly. Soon they returned saying, "I hadn't noticed that this was happening" and, "The prover didn't realize that these were proving symptoms."[14]

Apparently the provers cannot recognize their own symptoms; supervisors must prod, dig deep, and interpret. Another explanation is that there are no remedy-caused symptoms, and hence provers and supervisors alike must be encouraged to magnify the importance of perfectly ordinary symptoms so that they seem new and significant.

Sherr's discussion of meetings with all the provers is revealing:

These discussions help to trigger provers' memories for symptoms that they did not notice or were unsure about. So often provers and supervisors miss or disregard symptoms due to the subtle nature of provings, which may be as delicate as a mild breeze. For instance, in the Neon proving two provers experienced a delusion that someone was knocking on the door. When the symptom was mentioned a third prover recalled that they had the same experience during the proving, but had presumed that the kids were playing tricks. A fourth prover then related a dream of traveling around and knocking on people's doors before moving on. Of course one should closely investigate provers to ensure that these symptoms are not imaginary. However most homoeopaths are very conscientious about not fabricating symptoms. Those who still doubt the validity of reports could ask provers to swear on the Bible, as Hahnemann did. I have no doubt that without these group discussion[s] many valuable symptoms would be lost. They are essential for a good proving."[15]

Unfortunately for homeopathy, group discussions are a known way to create distorted or **false memories**. Swearing on the Bible might lessen conscious lying, but understanding the psychology of group pressure and the science of memory are even more important in preventing distorted data. Memories can feel real but not be based on a real event, and the person with the memory cannot perceive the falseness.[16]

Some of the early provings used significant doses of toxic materials[17] and the physical symptoms were surely caused biochemically by the ingested material. However, when these materials were diluted and potentized beyond any biochemical effect, and when innocuous materials (e.g., silica or food) and imponderables started to be proved, the eager provers kept on reporting symptoms. These reported effects could have been imagined symptoms created by expectations and false memories or real symptoms arising from normal events and normal health variability rather than symptoms caused by the remedies. Provings need to be conducted very carefully to sort out symptoms actually caused by the remedies from all the other symptoms people experience all the time.

Mental Associations of Remedies

The symptoms of many recently proved remedies seem to include what one might expect from invoking the doctrine of signatures (i.e., symptoms closely related to mental images of the material being proved). The following list shows examples of this in recent provings:

- Hecla lava is a remedy prepared from lava from Mt. Hecla in Iceland. Mental symptom includes "Very calm and poised person, but when provoked he used to burst into violent anger."[18]
- Taking Hydrogen produces "a great feeling of lightness and exhilaration followed by a profound sense of disconnectedness."[19]
- Provers testing Scorpion "developed tendencies of maliciousness and antisocial behavior and felt most comfortable in isolation."[20]
- Homeopath William Mann stated that the essence of the remedy Lac felinum (cat's milk) is "the conflict between dependence and independence. Namely, there is tension between the desire to give one's independence away for security or love and the equal urge to be on one's own under no one's power or subjugation."[21]

Four possible explanations come to mind to explain these close associations. (1) There were so many proving symptoms that by chance alone some would resemble common mental images of the remedy. Coincidences are probable given enough chances. (2) The provers knew what was being proved. (3) The material being proved was known to the researchers during the data extraction process; thus symptoms that fit the extractors' mental association were unconsciously given preference. (4) People who write about published provings certainly know what was proved and their preconceptions may color their interpretations.

It is clear that some homeopaths doing provings believe that the symptoms *should* be related to their impressions of the substance. The following excerpt is from the introductory comments to the proving report on Lava from Arizona by Misha Norland, a well-known homeopathic teacher, researcher, and practitioner:

> 1. The primary state of Lava is flowing and going; going for it no matter what; nothing gets in the way of an active Lava flow. This is a childlike state, which, if found in an adult, would obviously be viewed as their characteristic (forceful) predisposition.
>
> 2. The compensated, secondary state of Lava, is hardness (like the crust of cooling Lava), resistance and obstinacy. Both primary and secondary state may be viewed by others as unfeeling, the behavior as callus [*sic*] and amoral.
>
> 3. *The decompensated state is not brought out in the proving, yet we may expect that characteristic psychological components might be aridity and barrenness. Isolation.* [emphasis added][22]

Norland was in charge of this proving and so knew what was being proved. Not only is it probably that his vision of lava influenced many of the reported symptoms, but he even confidently noted symptoms, based on his notions of lava, that were not revealed in the proving (aridity, barrenness, and isolation).

If it is the remedies themselves that cure and cause symptoms, it would seem appropriate to let the remedies speak for themselves in provings.

Prover Sensitivity

For two centuries, homeopaths have noticed that not all provers get the same symptoms from the same remedy, and some get none at all. The homeopathic explanation is **sensitivity**: that not all provers are equally sensitive. An insensitive prover will get no symptoms from any remedy. Other provers might be sensitive to only one body part or health issue: "If we are proving Neon, each person will bring out a different symptomatology. One will bring out the throat, one will bring out the feet and one will bring out the mind. Thus the more varied the susceptibilities the more varied the symptoms."[23]

Some provers are especially sensitive only to one remedy, acquiring many and intense symptoms from it. Some are sensitive to all remedies. "A sensitive prover," says Sherr, "is a valuable asset to any proving. Some may enjoy the new experience and be willing to travel from proving to proving. As they are, naturally, the same person, the symptoms will appear to have a thread running through the provings. This does not invalidate these symptoms as they will always be a mix of the remedy and the constitution anyway."[24] This comment seems to suggest that the symptoms include some not caused by the remedy—that some symptoms are characteristic of the particular provers.

The sensitivity explanation for provers having different symptoms may seem plausible. To determine whether this explanation is valid, however, we need an independent measure of sensitivity, but there is none. In homeopathy, sensitive provers are defined as those who develop more symptoms in provings than others. Thus, the statement that sensitive people get more symptoms is just a definition of *sensitive*, not a testable hypothesis. A logically equivalent statement would be, "Children with demonstrated high academic achievement get high scores on academic achievement tests."

An alternative hypothesis for provers reacting differently is that the differences reflect the individual prover's health or personality regardless of the remedy. A prover who is thought to be especially good at revealing the digestive symptoms of a remedy may just have digestive problems. A prover who is thought to be especially good at revealing mental symptoms may just be mentally imaginative and expressive or unbalanced in some way.

Vithoulkas's description of provings is consistent with this hypothesis:

> Assuming that 50–100 provers participate in such an experiment, only the very rare subject will experience cure of preexisting symptoms, some will develop new symptoms within the first few days, another larger group will show symptoms after the twentieth day, and the majority will display only few or no symptoms at all during the entire period of observation. This wide variation in response is perfectly expectable from the variation in sensitivity. . . . Those who produce symptoms immediately are the most sensitive to the remedy.[25]

Vithoulkas's explanation sounds plausible, but so does an alternative. Suppose that a group of fifty to one hundred people was *not* given a homeopathic remedy, and the physical, mental, and emotional condition of the people was carefully observed for several months. People naturally get better, get worse, and develop new symptoms. One would almost certainly find that some develop new symptoms within the first twenty days and that more develop new symptoms after twenty days simply because that is a longer period (typical provings last several months). Many develop no new symptoms for the duration of the experiment either because they are generally healthier or because they are more objective in recognizing that most of their symptoms are "normal" or "natural" and hence should not be counted as having been caused by the remedy.

SENSITIVITY AND GENDER EQUITY

The following information on gender differences in homeopathy is offered without analysis. Something interesting may lie behind the numbers.

Jeremy Sherr does not find men and women equally valuable in provings: "[H]ypersensitivity is more common in women.... At the other end of the spectrum from the sensitives are those with lack of reaction, who will scarcely experience a sensation from any remedy. This tends to occur in a greater percentage in men. They are poor provers and difficult to cure."[26]

Many more practicing homeopaths are women than men, and many more students at homeopathic schools are female—the female percentages in both instances are typically between 75 and 95 percent.[27] Of the fifty-three students attending the three National Center for Homeopathy summer school courses in 2000, forty-six were female and seven were male. More homeopathic patients are female than male; in a recent survey of patients treated at the Liverpool Regional Department of Homeopathic Medicine, 75 percent of the patients were female.[28]

Peter Morrell, who provided some of the above statistics on women in homeopathy, has some speculation on and analysis of this issue.[29] His paper, "Gender in Homeopathy," is available online.

HOW PROVINGS SHOULD BE CONDUCTED

Many homeopaths believe that most provings are unassailably scientific. Homeopath Steven Cartwright states:

> Generally provings throughout the nineteenth century were conducted in a thorough and rigorous manner. The effects of preparations on groups of healthy volunteers were recorded faithfully, meticulously and objectively, with due and full regard to the volunteers' own words . . . without opinion or prior assumptions on the part of the observers. On the whole, provings are the one area of traditional homeopathic literature that is truly scientific.[30]

However, Wayne Jonas and Jennifer Jacobs comment: "By modern standards these experiments, or 'provings,' were not good science. Indeed, there was no blinding, no randomization, no placebos, no predetermined outcomes to be measured, no experiments on groups of sick individuals, no statistics or direct comparisons between groups of any kind."[31] Either we are lucky that Hahnemann and the other nineteenth-century provers got the right symptoms despite the lack of scientific procedures, or the tried-and-true homeopathic remedies in use today do not work in the manner that homeopaths think they do.

Many modern provings also lack the most elementary features to assure that the remedies are the causes of the reported symptoms. This view exists within as well as outside the homeopathic community. Commenting on many contemporary provings, homeopath Vithoulkas points out, "You record all the nonsense that goes on and the euphoria and the fantasy that goes on in the group and you record it as provings of the remedy. This is killing homeopathy at its very start."[32]

The following section explains how provings should be conducted to be consistent with modern scientific standards, assuming the objective is to determine which symptoms are caused by the remedies.

Control Group

In any group of people, whether the group is doing a proving or not, symptoms will arise and wane, particularly given the very broad homeopathic concept of *symptom*. Thus, when provers get a symptom, there is a chance that it was not caused by the remedy.

Standard techniques exist to determine whether the remedy is the cause. First, there must be a *control group*, which in this case would be composed of an equal number of similar people who are administered a fake remedy but otherwise are treated exactly the same as the test group. If approximately the same number of people in both groups get a particular symptom, then it is likely that the remedy being tested did not cause the symptom. Having such a control group would probably eliminate many of the ordinary symptoms listed by provers, such as fatigue, lower back pain, and scary dreams.

Most provings, old or recent, do not have true control groups. Most of the few provings that claim to have control groups use them for a different purpose, namely to try to keep everyone honest in reporting symptoms, which is considered more likely if some of the provers do not get the real remedy and none of the provers knows who has what.

Some provings use a control *time* rather than a control group. Participants are asked to record all their symptoms for some period, such as two weeks, before taking the remedy. This practice establishes a baseline of symptoms for comparison; any symptoms occurring after taking the remedy that also occurred before are excluded as not having been caused by the remedy. An even better approach is a blind crossover trial; all the provers are sometimes receiving the remedy and sometimes the placebo, but they do not know when they are getting which.

Number of Provers and Statistical Significance

If more treated than control people get a symptom, then mathematics can be used to calculate the odds of this occurrence happening by chance alone. If the odds that chance is the explanation are 1 in 20 or smaller, then the result is called statistically significant, and it is likely that the symptoms displaying **statistical significance** in the treated group were caused by the remedy.

Interestingly, many of the most knowledgeable and respected homeopathic researchers today reject the use of statistical significance. Jonas and Jacobs assert, "[T]he statistical approach only allows for crude symptoms to be examined because they must be grouped together and averaged in sufficient numbers. Unique and individual reactions to medications cannot easily be accounted for or included in this approach."[33] Clearly, homeopaths seem especially to value symptoms that only one or two provers exhibited. Sherr says, "Often the most important proving symptoms are brought mainly by one or two sensitive provers, the others serving to fill out the bulk of **common symptoms**" (emphasis added).[34] Yet these uncommon symptoms are the least likely to have been caused by the remedy precisely because only one or two provers had them; statistical significance is unlikely.

Obtaining statistically significant results is more likely with many provers. The number of provers used in provings over the last fifty years has usually been between ten and thirty; a few have had only one person and at least one had over one hundred. Most of the provings conducted more than a century ago had fewer than ten provers. Clinical trials of conventional medicines typically have hundreds or thousands of participants. The number of provers is so small in most cases that statistical significance appears not to be a consideration. What, then, is the rationale for the number chosen?

Sherr states:

I have often heard the opinion that a good proving needs a hundred or more provers. In my experience this number is far too large and will lead to an over-proved remedy. The danger here is overcrowding, with many common symptoms which will overload the repertory and inflate the remedy out of proportion to other remedies.

The other consideration is the enormous amount of time and work involved. . . . She [Anna Schadde] felt that 55 provers was too large a number and that in future they would use smaller groups. . . . Experience shows that 5 people will suffice for a small project, and that 15–20 will produce a very full remedy.[35]

Sherr asserts to the contrary, if the objective is to obtain complete and reliable symptoms for the remedy, having more provers is better; it should always increase the number of statistically significant conclusions and strengthen the confidence level in the conclusions. Yet, curiously, homeopaths feel that having too many provers decreases the usefulness of the data, producing "over-proved" remedies.

Homeopaths believe that different people have different sensitivities and hence bring out different aspects of the remedy. If so, how can five provers be enough? How can twenty be better than fifty?

But what if the provings data for each remedy are mostly just the random normal vicissitudes of human health? Provings with just a few provers would likely to produce a unique set of symptoms for each remedy just because people's normal symptoms are idiosyncratic and a few people do not exhibit all possible symptoms. With more and more provers involved, the symptoms would tend to represent the overall average distribution of natural symptoms, making remedies look similar and the job of finding the one most similar remedy more difficult. Perhaps for homeopaths, the optimum amount of proving data is enough to have sufficient variety to distinguish remedies from one another but not so much that the data are difficult to manage or that the remedies start to look just like each other. These objectives conflict with determining if the remedies *cause* the symptoms.

Blind and Double-Blind Procedures

In an ideal proving, the control group receives a look-alike but empty remedy (just a virgin sugar pill), which is usually called a **placebo**. However, if the participants know they have not received the real remedy, they will not expect to develop any symptoms, and this expectation can cause them not to get and not to report as many symptoms as other participants. Similarly, the knowledge that one has received the real remedy can cause more symptoms to arise. Thus no provers, whether or not they get the real remedy, must know whether they are in the treated or the control group. All the participants are then said to be *blind* or *masked*. This procedure removes a psychological difference between the groups.

Even with the participants being "blind," if the supervisors and anyone else who interacts with the provers knows which participants received the real remedy, their expectations and demeanor are involuntarily influenced, and patients can consciously or even unconsciously sense this influence and again develop more or fewer symptoms as a result. Such testing, then, needs to be **double blind**: Neither the provers nor any persons in contact with them must know who is in which group. Similarly, those who analyze the data for statistically significant differences between the groups must not know which group got the remedy and which got the placebo, to avoid possible bias.

Of course, someone needs to know, or all the effort is wasted. Therefore, at the beginning of such tests, someone puts the remedies and placebos in coded envelopes and records which codes correspond to real remedies and which to placebos. After all the data have been gathered and subjected to analysis, the researchers learn which group had which pill.

Provings should be blind in one extra sense; the provers should not interact with one another during the proving. In many provings, the provers live and work together since they are students at schools or attendees at workshops. This interaction can lead to a herding effect; by discussing their symptoms and experiences with one another, the participants may influence the symptoms and/or the reporting of the symptoms. The weaker members may tend to emulate the symptoms of the stronger members, leading to false statistical significance.[36]

No early provings were blind. Hahnemann used himself and his family and friends as provers, and he certainly knew what he was testing. The need for blinding was not recognized at that time. Sherr knows about blinding but seems to minimize its importance: "The double-blind test is supposed to compensate for bias in the observer and faith in the patient, but has never in fact been empirically tested or proved for either of these factors. It is notoriously difficult to enforce, as nurses and patients' relatives are both extraordinarily perceptive and in fact Coulter suggests that no medical double-blind tests have ever satisfied the requirements of a convincing trial."[37] Ignoring this aspect of testing almost guarantees bias in the results, and Sherr's view that double-blind procedures are unachievable is not shared by researchers in general.

Especially interesting is Sherr's opinion that there is no need for a blind control group to ascertain if the remedies cause symptoms because "Our long tradition of proving has served us well, mostly without the use of placebo!"[38] Sherr is saying good scientific methods are not needed because we homeopaths just know homeopathy works. Homeopaths may believe this, but the public deserves more and the conventional health-care community demands more.

Random Assignment of Provers

A subtle but important procedure is the **random assignment** of the volunteers to the treated and the placebo groups. If the treated group had mostly believers in homeopathy and the control group had mostly skeptics, any positive claims for the effectiveness of the remedy to induce symptoms would be suspect. Age, gender, medical history, lifestyle, personality, and factors of which no one is aware might influence the effect of the remedy. Thus good trials use a random process to determine which volunteers go into which group.

Duration of Observations

How long should provings last? For how long after taking a remedy can one expect to continue to have symptoms? In practice, most provings last from a few days to many months. The procedure for determining the endpoint of the longer provings is interesting. Vithoulkas says, "The subsequent observation period should be continued . . . until it is obvious that no more new symptoms are emerging."[39] Vithoulkas is assuming that the identification of new symptoms is clear and unambiguous; it is not.

In addition, scientists have found that having this kind of vague endpoint can lead to bias. The experiment might be terminated after the appearance of a particular group of symptoms, injecting a subjective element into the data. The results are more credible scientifically if the duration of the proving is stated in advance.

Dose Response

In tests of conventional medications, the treated group is usually further divided into a number of subgroups, each of which receives a different dose of the medication. This procedure satisfies the need to determine the amount of medication that is most effective for a cure and helps to quantify any side effects. Further, if there is no effect of dose on curing or side effects, then the whole test is cast into considerable doubt—if the amount of medication does not matter, then the medication itself must not matter.

The homeopathic interpretation of dose is different. In homeopathy the amount of the remedy taken is thought to be relatively unimportant compared to the number of times the remedy is taken, the time between doses, and the potency (chapter 6). Thus there are a number of parameters that might represent the homeopathic surrogate for dose.[40]

Provings rarely if ever investigate the effect of the amount of remedy taken; typically one pellet is consumed each time. Nor do they investigate the effect of the number of times the remedy is taken or the interval between doses. Many provings involve taking the remedy just once and then observing any response. Others may involve taking the remedy up to six times over a few days, or three times a day for up to a month. In all cases of such repetitive dosing, the prover stops taking the remedy as soon as symptoms believed to be caused by the remedy are apparent. However, no attempt is made to measure different responses to differing procedures. The only objective is to start the proving reaction in the provers, and then to stop giving the remedy.

Provings also rarely investigate the effect of potency. Some provings use only a single potency; others involve multiple potencies. Sherr asserts that the potencies used in provings are not critical: "In my provings, I have used a wide range of potencies—6C, 15C, 30C, 200C. It is equally valid to use one potency only, say 30C, or a single dose of 1M [100C]."[41] Vithoulkas, in contrast, advocates careful exploration of potency using three separate provings, the first using **molecular doses** from 1X to 12X, depending on toxicity; the second using 30C potency; and the final using 10,000 or 50,000C. Fifty to one hundred provers participate in the first proving, but only those who exhibit symptoms quickly in the first proving participate in the next two provings. The higher potency provings are thought by some homeopaths to bring out the subtler symptoms, especially the mental and emotional symptoms. The whole process takes well over a year; very few provings have been done this way, and consequently very few repertories or materia medicae include potency-specific symptoms. Overall, provings rarely provide information on the response to dose, however "homeopathic dose" is interpreted.

Summary and Conclusion

Most provers are undoubtedly honest and sincere in reporting their symptoms, but the question is whether the symptoms were caused by the remedy or by something else. Symptom causes other than the remedy might include the following:

- The symptoms of the provers are the normal symptoms one would expect in any group of people over a few months, due to diet, chronic health conditions, newly contracted illnesses or injuries, allergies, exercise, stress, sleep, aging, environment, and work.
- Provers may unconsciously imagine or enhance symptoms in an effort to please their supervisors or to fulfill their own expectations.
- False memories of symptoms can be created through interactions among the provers and their supervisors. Some people can be convinced, or can convince themselves, that they remember something that never happened.
- Some provers may be truly psychosomatic, constantly (with or without a homeopathic remedy) perceiving and reporting symptoms that have no cause other than their own psyches.
- Even if the supervisors and director do not know what remedy is being tested, they may bias the selection of data once they formulate an idea about the remedy picture.
- There may be a herding effect. If the provers communicate with one another during the proving or data analysis afterward, one or more members may influence the group, thus skewing the data.

Provings rarely use the double-blind, placebo-controlled random-assignment procedures and criteria for statistical significance, all of which are signs of high methodological quality; they are designed to filter out the symptom origins just listed, leaving only those caused by the remedy. In fact, the homeopathic procedures typically encourage false positives and put special value on statistically insignificant strange, rare, and peculiar symptoms.

Perhaps the most sobering evidence is a study by Flávio Dantas and Peter Fisher of all provings published in the United Kingdom between 1945 and 1995.[42] The authors categorized forty-five studies by their methodological quality and found that the lowest-quality studies reported many symptoms as having been caused by the remedies, whereas *the highest-quality studies found zero symptoms related to the remedy* (figure 4.2). The symptoms seem to disappear when the methodology assures that the symptoms come only from the remedies. The researchers conclude, "Our systematic review has shown that some recent provings lack adequate control and analysis; the results of such studies are unreliable and may be positively misleading and damaging to both homeopathy and to patients."[43]

Harald Walach and Wayne Jonas also were not impressed by the quality of most provings: "The few HPT's [provings] which explicitly addressed the question of whether symptoms observed with a homeopathic remedy are different from placebo were not successful in demonstrating a difference."[44] In a recent double-blind study by Vickers,[45] professional homeopaths were either given a homeopathic remedy (Bryonia 12C) or a placebo, and were asked to decide which they had received by observing their own proving symptoms. Fifty participants completed the study. Chance would yield an average of twenty-five correct responses; there were twenty-eight correct responses in the study, not a statistically significant result. In a recent (2001) high-quality proving, Walach and his colleagues concluded, "There is no indication that Belladonna 30CH[46] produces symptoms different from placebo or from no intervention. Symptoms of a homeopathic pathogenetic trial (HTP) are most likely chance fluctuations."[47] All these studies suggest that homeopathic remedies do not cause symptoms in healthy individuals.

Homeopaths tend to mistake meticulous effort for substance. Most proving supervisors take pride in careful data documentation; dates and times for all symptoms are written down and sometimes recordings are made of interviews, so that accuracy can be checked later. But the key question is not the existence of the provers' symptoms or the accuracy of reporting, but whether the symptoms were actually caused by the remedy.

In all fields of science, confidence in results rises substantially if the results are replicated by different investigators. There are very few if any quality provings with quality replication attempts. Homeopaths do not generally feel the need for reprovings; their cured cases convince them that their provings data are valid.

The information presented in this chapter makes the validity of provings look bleak. It does not help that some of today's most noted provers seem to dismiss good methodology as either impossible to achieve, unnecessary, or even detrimental. Even the ultimate authority in the United States on homeopathic remedies and provings, the HPUS, explicitly belittles the importance of quality methodology:

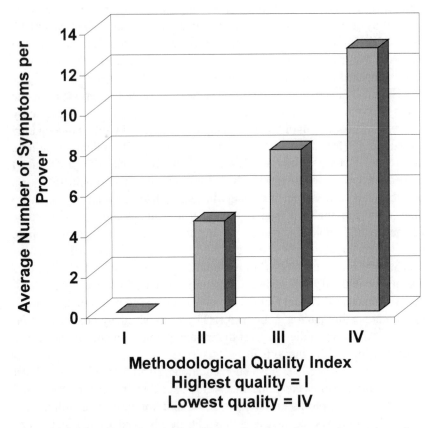

Figure 4.2. The effect of methodological quality of provings on the number of symptoms. The highest quality studies have the least symptoms attributed to the remedy. (Data from Dantas and Fisher, 1998)

There are still other points arising from contemporary research methods which should be taken into consideration as well: the issue of placebo control, the selection of volunteers by means of medical standard criteria, and the availability of clearly defined scales for the assessment of symptoms. These aspects may be respected in the planning of modern homeopathic drug provings; *however, their presence or absence should not be used to disqualify a homeopathic drug proving strictly done according to the directions set forth by Hahnemann* [emphasis added].[48]

This statement makes it clear that tradition is more important to homeopaths than sound procedures.

Homeopaths' internal reality is that proving symptoms are caused by the remedies. This internal reality, originating from the provings themselves, is reinforced by tradition, training, and the practice of homeopathy wherein patients are seen to improve when given remedies whose symptoms are based primarily on provings. The internal perception is that the provings *must* be valid. Yet, the external reality does not support this internal reality.

NOTES

1. Elizabeth Loftus, "Creating False Memories," *Scientific American* 277, no. 3 (1997): 70–75.

2. Flávio Dantas and Peter Fisher, "A Systematic Review of Homeopathic Pathogenic Trials ('Provings') Published in the United Kingdom from 1945 to 1995," in *Homeopathy: A Critical Appraisal*, ed. Edzard Ernst and Eckhart G. Hahn (Woburn, Mass.: Butterworth-Heinemann, 1998), pp. 69–97.

3. Jeremy Sherr, *The Dynamics and Methodology of Homeopathic Provings* (Malvern, U.K.: Dynamis Books, 1995), p. 72.

4. Ibid.

5. Ibid., p. 70.

6. Samuel Hahnemann, *Materia Medica Pura*, vol. 2 (1817; reprint, New Delhi: B. Jain Publishers, 1999), pp. 270–83.

7. Misha Norland, "The Homeopathic Proving of Basaltic Lava" [online], http://www.hominf.org/lava/lavafr.htm [Nov. 29, 2002].

8. Examples of nonspecific times are morning, afternoon, dusk, and night.

9. James Tyler Kent, *Repertory of the Homeopathic Materia Medica* (1897–99; reprint, New Delhi: B. Jain Publishers, 1999), pp. 133–35.

10. George Vithoulkas, *The Science of Homeopathy* (New York: Grove Press, 1980), p. 145.

11. Sherr, p. 22.

12. See, for instance, Abdur Rehman, *Encyclopedia of Remedy Relationships in Homeopathy* (Heidelberg: Karl F. Haug Verlag, 1997).

13. Sherr, pp. 41–42.

14. Ibid., pp. 46–47.

15. Ibid., p. 66.

16. Loftus.

17. Paul Herscu, *Provings Volume, with a Proving of Alcoholus* (Amherst, Mass.: New England School of Homeopathy Press, 2002), p. 137.

18. Frans Vermeulen, *Synoptic Materia Medica 2* (Haarken, Netherlands: Merlijn Publishers, 1998), pp. 431–32.

19. Robert Ullman and Judyth Reichenberg-Ullman, *The Patient's Guide to Homeopathic Medicine* (Edmonds, Wash: Picnic Point Press, 1995), p. 45.

20. Ibid.

21. Quoted in Evann Wilcosky, "Lac Felinum, Report on a Presentation by William Mann," *Homeopathy Today* 20, no. 9 (2000): 28.

22. Norland, "The Homeopathic Proving of Basaltic Lava," [Nov. 28, 2002].

23. "Similia for Windows 95," (software), (Nottingham, U.K.: Miccant Ltd).

24. Sherr, p. 25.

25. Vithoulkas, p. 152.

26. Sherr, pp. 24, 26.

27. Peter Morrell, "Gender in Homeopathy," paper presented to the Conference on the History of Unconventional Medicine, University of Linköping, Sweden, Sept. 10–12, 1998. Available online at http://homeoint.org/morrell/articles/pm_gende.htm [Nov. 29, 2002].

28 W. R. Richardson, "Patient Benefit Survey: Liverpool Regional Department of Homeopathic Medicine," *British Homeopathic Journal* 90 (2001): 158–62.

29. Morrell.

30. Steven Cartwright, "A Re-examination of Homeopathic Philosophy and a Simplified Approach to Practice," *Homeopath* 84 (2002): 17.

31. Wayne Jonas and Jennifer Jacobs, *Healing with Homeopathy: The Doctors' Guide* (New York: Warner Books, 1996), p. 28.

32. George Vithoulkas, "A Man with a Mission: Interview with George Vithoulkas," *Homoeopathic Links* 12, no. 4 (1999): 204.

33. Jonas and Jacobs, p. 28.

34. Sherr, p. 25.

35. Ibid., p. 45.

36. Clinical trials of conventional drugs seldom involve this problem because the participants usually do not know or interact with one another.

37. Sherr, p. 36.

38. Ibid., p. 37.

39. Vithoulkas, *The Science of Homeopathy*, p. 152.

40. In this book and in virtually all health-care contexts except homeopathy, dose means the amount of a therapeutic agent to be taken at one time. In homeopathy, dose means *all* the details around taking the remedy—the potency, the physical form (pills or drops), any additional dilution, stirring or shaking to be done by the patient, and the number and timing of any repeats (for example, twice per day for four days).

41. Sherr, p. 56.

42. Dantas and Fisher, pp. 69–97.

43. Ibid., p. 95.

44. Harald Walach and Wayne B. Jonas, "Homeopathy," in *Clinical Research in Complementary Therapies*, ed. George Lewith, Wayne B. Jonas, and Harald Walach (London: Churchill Livingstone, 2002), p. 239.

45. A. Vickers et al., "Can Homeopaths Detect Homeopathic Medicines? A Pilot Study for a Randomized, Double-Blind, Placebo-Controlled Investigation of the Proving Hypothesis," *British Homeopathic Journal* 90, no. 3 (2001): 126–30.

46. The "H" in "30CH" indicates that the remedy was prepared using the Hahnemannian as opposed to Korsakovian method. See appendix 1.

47. Harald Walach et al., "The Effects of Homeopathic Belladonna 30CH in Healthy Volunteers: A Randomized, Double-Blind Experiment," *Journal of Psychosomatic Research* 50 (2001): 155–60.

48. *The Homeopathic Pharmacopoeia of the United States, Abstracts: 2001* (HPUS) (Washington, D.C.: Homeopathic Pharmacopoeia Convention of the United States, 2001), p. 14.

5. *Selecting the Remedy*

Once the patient's symptoms have been assessed, the appropriate remedy is selected as the one that best covers the symptoms. On the surface, this process sounds like it would lead most homeopaths to prescribe the same remedy for the same patient. However, such consistency seems unlikely given the many different schools and subschools of homeopathy. As homeopath Todd Rowe notes, "There are as many ways to analyze a case as there are homeopaths to analyze them [it]. The methods range from a complex computerized analysis to dowsing, from a deep, essence-level understanding of the person to prescribing based on pathology."[1]

Does it matter if homeopaths do not agree on the remedy? Perhaps any of a number of remedies works equally well; perhaps there is not just one simillimum. This possibility also brings up the question of how good a match is needed between remedy and patient. And if a great many remedies work equally well, perhaps the remedy itself is not part of the health benefit. These issues will be discussed toward the end of this chapter.

THE PROCESS

The variety of approaches used by self-declared homeopaths to select remedies is very large; even within classical homeopathy, the number is substantial.

Factors influencing the choice of a remedy by classical homeopaths include (see appendix 5 for more details):

- The nature and thoroughness of the homeopath's case taking; not all homeopaths elicit the same symptoms
- The homeopath's selection and grading of the most important symptoms from the case taking
- The homeopath's choice of which repertory to use
- The grading of the remedies listed under each symptom; some remedies are thought to have a stronger association than others with each particular symptom
- The relative value the homeopath places on strange, rare, and peculiar symptoms
- In a multiple approach, the homeopath's decision concerning which combination of the above procedures to use and what relative importance to give to each
- The homeopath's study of the *gestalt* of the remedy to assess its fit with the patient's essence

Additional factors that are not always considered part of classical homeopathy include (additional details in appendix 5):

- The homeopath's decision on whether or not to give extra weight to **small remedies,** or to exclude **large remedies** or **polycrests** (remedies with a large number of symptoms)
- The decision to use or avoid remedies belonging to particular remedy families, classes, or rows and columns in the periodic table, or associated with particular elements in the periodic table
- The decision to prescribe a constitutional remedy rather than a remedy based on symptoms of the patient's illness
- The decision on whether to use patient symptoms directly or to abstract from the symptoms a general theme or "central delusion"
- The emphasis or lack thereof on *etiology* (the perceived cause of the symptoms)
- The decision to use or not to use the doctrine of signatures

- The decision on whether to treat only the chief complaint instead of the whole person
- The judgment on whether the patient is compensating for his mental and emotional symptoms and hence making them difficult for the homeopath to perceive
- The awareness of cultural differences that can be mistaken for symptoms
- The decision to treat one perceived layer of disease rather than the patient's total symptom picture
- The decision to use such nonclassical methods as electrodiagnosis, dowsing, or applied kinesiology
- The extent to which the homeopath uses *remedy relationships*—remedies that are *complementary, inimical, antidotal, collateral, intercurrent,* or that *follow well* (see appendix 5)

Clearly, choosing the remedy is not a well-defined procedure that a computer could be programmed to follow. Individual judgment and completely different philosophies pervade the process. In this sense, selecting the remedy is an art, not a science; it is inevitable that not all homeopaths will agree on the same remedy for the same case.

CONSISTENCY TESTING

Most studies on the consistency of homeopathic prescribing have been negative. A recent test involved a patient who had been given two homeopathic remedies; subsequent improvement of the patient convinced the homeopath that both remedies were "correct." As an experiment, three experienced homeopaths later watched a videotape of the case taking and selected what they thought were the appropriate remedies. None of them selected the "correct" remedies.[2]

In another recent study, twenty-seven homeopaths analyzed a paper case (the symptoms from the case taking had been written down). Two-thirds selected the "wrong" remedy, and there were fourteen different "wrong" answers.[3] The results would have been even more inconsistent had the test been more realistic. Paper cases necessarily include data selection and interpretation, and the practitioner in this case had already selected certain symptoms as being especially important. A more realistic test would require the homeopaths to start with all the raw data, or even to conduct their own separate interviews with the patient.[4]

Some homeopaths acknowledge this problem: "Why is it," asks Divya Chhabra, "that we can have five homeopaths in a room, all observing the same patient, and yet have five different suggestions of remedies? Because each homeopath sees a different expression of the patient."[5] Joseph Zarfaty says, "We all know that when homeopaths meet to discuss a case, they rarely decide on the same remedy."[6]

Is conventional medicine consistent in its prescriptions? No, but it is probably more so than homeopathy. One of conventional medicine's advantages is its recognition of diseases, for each of which there are typically only a few appropriate medicines, whereas in homeopathy there are hundreds of possible remedies because of the importance placed on individual idiosyncratic and nondisease symptoms.

OBSESSION WITH *THE* SIMILLIMUM

Homeopaths in general work hard to find the *one* remedy whose symptoms best match those of the patient—the simillimum. As Constantine Hering puts it, "We [try] our best to find the most similar among all of our drugs, the only one that [will] cure."[7] Most other health-care practitioners recognize that any of a few medicines or treatments might do the job.

The concern for a unique remedy has resulted in some procedures that differ from those of almost all other health-care practitioners. Some of these procedures can be interpreted as having no justification other than to narrow down the choice of remedies, increasing the chances of having a single remedy stand out at the end.

For instance, homeopaths value the patients' verbal descriptions of symptoms more than more objective laboratory measures. It does not usually matter to the patient or to a physician whether the pain from corns is aching, burning, pinching, pressing, pulsating, shooting, stinging, or tearing. However, each of these descriptions points to a different homeopathic remedy, helping homeopaths narrow the choice down to a single remedy.

Similarly, homeopaths want to know everything that makes symptoms feel better or worse. Is it important to the patient or to understanding the medical condition if headaches tend to start at 9:00 or 9:30 A.M., or might this information just be a way to narrow the choice of remedies?

Even more important to a homeopath are mental and emotional symptoms. Luc De Schepper states, "The patient's disease symptoms come *last* in the priority."[8] George Vithoulkas agrees: "Mental symptoms are the most important in selecting a medicine."[9] Why? One interpretation is that without these symptoms, selecting a *single* best remedy would be much more difficult. Many provers for many remedies report similar aches and pains, but the mental and emotional symptoms tend to be unique; fewer people have identically reported dreams than identically reported sore throats.

As previously stated, homeopathy puts high value on strange, rare, and peculiar symptoms. Vithoulkas says, "In . . . complex cases, it may be necessary to 'throw out' even important mental or general symptoms and to rely on seemingly less significant but more peculiar symptoms."[10] Again, why? Such symptoms are not usually seen as relevant by a patient and are the least likely to have been caused by the remedy in a proving. Some of the symptoms are very strange indeed, for example, "painful erections when traveling on railroad cars, excepting when [the patient] found himself obliged to enter conversation."[11] Perhaps these symptoms are valuable to homeopaths because, like mental and emotional symptoms, they narrow the choice of remedies.

Homeopaths also do not want too many people participating in provings. With more provers, remedies will have more symptoms in common, again making it harder to find a single remedy, despite the fact that in scientific research, having more data is always better.

Thus, it can be argued that the most pressing concern of the patient (the chief complaint), and objectivity have both been relegated to the back seat in favor of narrowing the treatment down to a single remedy.

How Close Is Close Enough?

If only one remedy can do the job, how closely must that remedy match the patient's symptoms to be effective? Is the effect proportional to the closeness of the remedy? For some patients, might there be no proven remedy sufficiently close to their symptoms to be the simillimum?

Homeopaths seem to believe that in an ideal world the simillimum's symptoms should include *all* of the patient's symptoms. If a symptom that is not in the remedy picture disappears during treatment, it is presumed to belong to the remedy. For instance, in a recently reported case,[12] the patient's symptoms seemed to call for Pulsatilla except that the remedy picture for Pulsatilla did not include the patient's symptom, "zigzags before the eyes." When the zigzags cleared after the patient took Pulsatilla, this improvement was taken as evidence that eye zigzags were in fact cured by

Pulsatilla. Homeopaths would say that the remedy pictures in materia medicae do not cover all of a patient's symptoms for a number of reasons: (1)
the remedy pictures are incomplete or have errors, (2) the case taking has
errors, and (3) not all potential remedies have been proved. They acknowledge that for these reasons a simillimum may be hard to discover, but they
do not doubt its existence.

   If perfect matching of the remedy to the symptoms is not possible, how
close is close enough? In its infancy, homeopathy had only a few remedies
from which to choose (see table 5.1). With such a limited selection of remedies, the matches were often not very close; either there must have been very
few cures or else this early success is evidence that the match need not be
very close. Since homeopathy's developers were not discouraged from continuing, it seems more likely that the match did not need to be very close.

Table 5.1. Historical Trend in the Number of Available Remedies

Date	Number of Remedies	Source	
		Author	Title
1805	27	Hahnemann	*Fragmenta de Viribus Medicamentorum Positivis Sive in Sano Corpore Humano Observatis*
1811–1821	67	Hahnemann	*Materia Medica Pura*
1897–1899	about 600	Kent	*Repertory of the Homeo-pathic Materia Medica*
2003	about 1,300		HPUS
2003	over 2,000		Helios[a] pharmacy and Synthesis[b] repertory

   a. Remedy List, Helios Homoeopathic Pharmacy [online], http://www.helios.co.uk
[Nov. 2002].
   b. *Synthesis Eight for Radar* (Assesse, Belgium: Archibel, 2002).

   Currently, with over 1,300 remedies officially recognized by the HPUS
and a few times this number in use, and with computers to help search for
symptoms in materia medicae, homeopathy should be working better than
ever.[13] It should be easier now to pick an effective remedy since so many
more are close enough, or cures should be better (faster or longer lasting)

because it is possible to get a much closer match between patient and remedy. Yet the success rate for homeopathy has not increased. There are no hard data on historical trends in cure rates, mostly because the evidence is almost entirely anecdotal. However, the self-reported cure rate from experienced practitioners seems always to have been around 70 to 80 percent.

Most homeopaths believe that the match is more critical when the potency is higher. Thus, another possible explanation for homeopathy's early success despite the small number of remedies available is that lower potencies were used then (remedies were less dilute).

Homeopaths often suggest that the remedy must be the best *available* fit to the patient's symptoms, not necessarily a very close fit. Yasgur's *Homeopathic Dictionary* defines the simillimum as "the remedy that most closely corresponds to the totality of symptoms . . . and when found, is always curative (or in incurable cases, it is the best possible palliative remedy)."[14] This definition is consistent with the apparent constancy of homeopathic effectiveness as remedies have been added over the last two centuries. However, since the number of available remedies has increased so much, the best-fit remedy in Hahnemann's time might not be the best today for the same patient; presumably there is now a remedy that is a better fit. Would only today's better-fitting remedy work on a patient alive today, even though a less well-matched remedy did the job a century or two ago? It would indeed be peculiar if the power of a remedy to cure a patient could be quenched by human knowledge about other remedies.

CONCLUSION

Does it matter, even within classical homeopathy, that different remedies are prescribed by different homeopaths? Maybe most of the remedies come close enough to matching the patient's symptom picture that a cure will be achieved anyway. If finding the single closest remedy is not considered critical for most patients, then the remedy perhaps should not be called "*the* simillimum," because there is not just one.

However, a glance at the titles of articles in homeopathic journals and magazines makes it clear that most homeopaths see each case as related to and hence cured by a single remedy. The following list of all the titles of articles related to cases in the spring 2001 issue of *Homoeopathic Links*, a journal of classical homeopathy, illustrates this tendency.

- I Want to Become a Hitler and a Mother Theresa: A Case of Veratrum Album
- I Want to Be Remembered like Mahatma Gandhi: A Case of Veratrum Album
- Is Everyone Telling Me the Truth?: A Case of Ruta Graveolens
- Treating "Silver Baby": A Case of Griscelli's Syndrome
- I Want a Reputation from Myself: A Case of Bryonia Alba
- I Do Not Care to Live: A Case of Lac Defloratum
- Delusion Young, She Is: A Case of Ginseng
- I'm a Sinner. I'm Stuck . . . : A Case of Thuja
- Shocked by the Conditions in India: An Indication for Aloe
- The Tailed Jay: A Case and a Proving of Graphium Agamemnon
- A Guide to the Muse: A Case of Apeira Syringaria
- Hypothyroidism: A Case of Bufo Rana
- The Tall Nervous Flyer: A Case of Hyperthyroidism

Most homeopaths do not believe that prescribing is inconsistent. Their belief that most homeopaths would prescribe the same remedy for the same case comes from *retrospective* understanding of others' prescriptions. Homeopaths always have reasons for their particular remedy selection—reasons that usually make sense to other homeopaths—but that is very different from selecting the same remedy in the first place. Nonetheless, these retrospective reasons contribute to homeopaths' internal reality that they agree and consequently would score well in consistency testing.

If prescribing is inconsistent and yet most homeopaths experience approximately the same cure rates with their patients, the cures must be independent of the particular remedies used, and the remedies themselves may not contribute to the cures.

NOTES

1. Todd Rowe, *Homeopathic Methodology* (Berkeley: North Atlantic Books, 1998), p. 101.

2. Judyth Reichenberg-Ullman et al., Case Analysis Roundtable: Common Threads of Success," *Simillimum* 9 (1996): 22–41.

3. M. Aghadiuno, "A Study of the Inter-observer Reliability of Paper Case Analysis," *Homeopathy* (formerly *British Homeopathic Journal*) 91, no. 1 (2002): 10–17. The paper states that twenty-seven practitioners were involved, but lists twenty-eight first-choice remedies. Thus the "two-thirds" may be not quite correct.

4. Should testing for consistent remedy selection involve a common inter-

view (case taking) or separate interviews? Homeopaths have distinct personalities and interview styles that will elicit a different mix of symptoms from the same patient, possibly contributing to the selection of different remedies. For this reason, one could argue that separate interviews should be part of any test. However, it could also be argued that the patient's condition changes with time, and therefore the consistency *should* be based on a common interview. A thorough test of reproducibility might require both approaches.

5. Divya Chhabra, as quoted in Penny Edwards, "Finding the Innermost State Through the Circle: Inspiration and Compelling Teaching from Divya Chhabra," *Homeopath* 84 (2002): 6.

6. Joseph Zarfaty, "Homeopathy and the Search for Meaning," *Homoeopathic Links* 15, no. 2 (2002): 80.

7. Constantine Hering, quoted in Harris Coulter, *Divided Legacy* (Berkeley: North Atlantic Books, 1982), p. 337.

8. Luc De Schepper, *Hahnemann Revisited* (Santa Fe: Full of Life Publishing, 2001), p. 5.

9. George Vithoulkas, *The Science of Homeopathy* (New York: Grove Press, 1980), p. 216.

10. Ibid., p. 212.

11. Coulter, p. 338.

12. Example taken from Sandra M. Chase, "Homeopathy for Serious Physical Pathology," *Homeopathy Today* 22, no. 1 (2002): 26.

13. It might also be argued that high cure rates are more difficult to attain today because our bodies face more challenges due, for instance, to more chemicals in the environment. This is an interesting proposition and is popularly held to be true. Yet death rates for most types of cancer have been steady or declining over the last few decades, and life expectancies have risen substantially over the last two centuries. These facts suggest some combination of a more healthful environment and better health care.

14. Jay Yasgur, *Homeopathic Dictionary* (Greenville, Penn.: Van Hoy Publishers, 1998), p. 234.

6. *Administering the Remedy*

T he homeopath's job is not finished once the remedy has been chosen. Most remedies are available in many different potencies in each of the three different scales (X, C, and LM), and in liquid and various solid forms. Moreover, the homeopath must decide how much remedy the patient should take, how many times it should be taken, and at what time intervals. Another complication is the intricate procedures for taking remedies, the relevance of which is unclear. Homeopaths also believe that many environmental factors can deactivate stored remedies. Thus the process does not end with selection of the remedy.

SELECTING THE POTENCY

Homeopathic remedies are available in a huge range of potencies from 1X to over 100,000C. Differences of opinion exist as to how to select the best potency. Some books say very little, while some say a lot. Most authors say that potency is not critical. Dana Ullman states that for acute ailments, "Once one finds the correct remedy, most potencies of it will have a beneficial effect, with the best potency simply having a deeper and/or faster result."[1] Will Taylor comments, "Most of our patients could be successfully treated with just about any dosing method we wish to throw at them—crude dose, tinctures, low decimal [X] doses, high centesimals [C], dry centesimals in repetition, LMs in careful management, whatever."[2] Many homeopaths do not believe there is much difference between X and C remedies; they think that 12C and 12X are approximately equivalent, despite a difference in dilution by a factor of one trillion.

Nonetheless, potency is believed to make some difference. Definitions of low and high potencies vary but roughly are as indicated in table 6.1.

Table 6.1. Potency Ranges	
Low	Up to 30C
Medium	30C to 1000C
High	Above 1000C

Source: Julie Bernard, *Potency in Homeopathic Prescribing* (Mill Valley, Calif.: self-published, 1999), p. 12.

Homeopaths have many reasons for preferring lower or higher potencies (see table 6.2). Some of these reasons appear to be contradictory.

Table 6.2. Guidelines for Selecting Potency	
Low Potency	**High Potency**
Best for self-prescribing	Only professional should prescribe
Appropriate for acute conditions	More suited for chronic or mental/emotional conditions
Appropriate when "the illness is chronic or slow"[a]	More suited when "the illness is acute or sudden"[c]
Needed in cases of advanced pathology and incurable cases[b]	Appropriate "in serious cases, acute or chronic"[d]
Appropriate when patient's susceptibility is high	Appropriate "where the symptoms are especially intense and well-marked"[e]
Short-lived effects—frequent repetitions often needed	Longer lasting effects—less frequent or no repetitions needed

Does not require as close a match between patient's and remedy's symptoms	The remedy must be more accurate; if one misses the simillimum by just a little, there will be no cure, or the patient may get worse in some way as part of the cure, or there will be an inadvertent proving
Appropriate if patient is old, has weak vital force or weak constitution, is sensitive	Appropriate if patient is young, has strong vital force or strong constitution
Appropriate if patient is being exposed to **antidoting** substances	
	Deeper-acting, more likely to influence mental and emotional realms. Useful "in chronic cases, when the illness is directly traceable to something that happened long ago."[f]

a. Timothy Dooley, "Choosing the Right Remedy Dosage," *Homeopathy Today* 21, no. 11 (2001): 32–33.
b. Luc De Schepper, *Hahnemann Revisited* (Santa Fe: Full of Life Publishing, 2001), p. 52.
c. Dooley, p. 32.

d. Richard Moskowitz, *Resonance: The Homeopathic Point of View* (http://www. Xlibris.com, Xlibris Corporation, 2000), p. 67.
e. Ibid.
f. Ibid.

Some homeopaths think that if the same potency of a remedy is given repeatedly to a patient, the patient becomes less sensitive to that potency. This problem can be overcome by switching to a higher potency. Thus, a patient may be given ever-higher potencies as the treatment progresses.

Still other homeopaths see even more complexity in choosing potencies. Elizabeth Wright-Hubbard found it effective in sluggishly responding cases to switch from the common potencies such as 10,000C, 50,000C, and 100,000C to an irregular potency of, say, 47,000C. "This change seems to start a new rhythm or cycle, . . . as though the vital force became bored with the decimal system and responded with a renewed spurt to the alteration of potency."[3]

Some practitioners claim that a few particular potencies (such as 6, 12, 24, and 200, both X and C) "are gentler on the vital force and do not cause severe aggravations or aggravate at all."[4] (An **aggravation** is getting worse as a part of getting better. See chapter 7.) Some experiments on nonhumans suggest that different sets of potencies are particularly strong, such as dilutions of 15, 25, 45, 65, 94, and 110X.[5]

Some homeopaths believe that LM remedies (wherein each dilution is a factor of 50,000) may be the best, offering high strength with little aggravation.

It is difficult to comment on the choice of potency. There seems to be no clear theoretical structure on which to base the choice, and there certainly are no scientifically based data on the consequences of the choice. Most homeopaths stress the need to individualize potency for each specific patient, but the number of supposedly relevant parameters and their vagueness virtually guarantees little agreement among homeopaths. The parameters affecting individualization of potency include the condition of the vital force; the patient's susceptibility, sensitivity, and temperament; interfering factors; the pace of the illness; and above all else, the patient's responses.[6]

Some combination remedies seem to sidestep the question of which potency is best by including many potencies. For instance, the remedy Apis-Homaccord[7] in its oral drop form contains Apis mellifica in potencies of 2X, 10X, 30X, 200X, and 1,000X—the right and wrong potency for every situation. Perhaps the manufacturers hope that the body will select the most appropriate potency and ignore the ones that are inappropriate.

If the active ingredient is the original medicinal molecules or water clusters, then it is pointless to mix potencies. It is like mixing ground up iron ore of low and high grades and then claiming that the mix has the properties of both; it doesn't—it has properties of an intermediate grade ore—it is an average.

WHY ISN'T POTENCY MORE CRITICAL?

Homeopathic potency is a concept without a parallel in conventional or herbal medicine. There is no way to measure a remedy's strength for remedies past the molecular limits of about 12C and 24X. There is not even a laboratory method to verify that any such remedy is in fact the remedy it claims to be; all such remedies in all potencies are indistinguishable from plain sugar pills using any known scientific method.

Homeopathy has no quantitative models for remedy strength. Nonetheless, it is instructive to speculate on how the strength of a remedy depends on its potency. Four of many possible mathematical models are discussed here, chosen to represent a very wide range of possibilities.

1. Remedy strength increases in proportion to dilution—a 2C remedy is one hundred times stronger than a 1C remedy because it is one hundred times more dilute.
2. Each dilution and succussion increases remedy strength by a factor of two; thus a 2C remedy is twice as strong as a 1C remedy, and a 3C remedy is twice as strong as a 2C remedy.
3. Each dilution and succussion step increases remedy strength by 1 percent. Thus a 2C remedy is 1 percent stronger than a 1C remedy.
4. The remedy strength is related to the C number; either the ratio of the C numbers represents the ratio of the remedy strengths, or the difference in C numbers is the ratio of remedy strengths. This latter model is mathematically inconsistent, but might represent an approximation of some people's impression of remedy strength.

How much difference is there between a 12C and a 30C remedy? Based on model 1, the 30C is a trillion trillion trillion times stronger than a 12C (see table 6.3). Models 2 and 3 give 260,000 times stronger and 20 percent stronger respectively for a 30C compared to a 12C remedy. Models 1 and 2 give such large differences that they must be incorrect since homeopaths see 12C and 30C potencies as nearly equivalent. Model 3 yields such a small difference that 12C and 30C remedies would be nearly indistinguishable, which is closer to how homeopaths use them. However, model 3 predicts that a 20,000C remedy should be more than 10^{43} times stronger than a 10,000C remedy: that's ten million billion billion billion times stronger! If any of these three models is anywhere near correct, differences in strength of more than a factor of a trillion must not be critical since in-between strength remedies are rarely used.

Homeopaths do not see a need for all potencies. A representative remedy kit for professional homeopaths might consist of 30, 200, 1,000, and 10,000C potencies. Grocery and drug store (single) remedies for the self-prescriber are typically sold in potencies of 6, 12, and 30X and/or C.

	Model 1 Strength Proportional to Amount of Dilution	Model 2 Strength Doubles with Each Dilution	Model 3 Strength Increases by 1% with Each Dilution	Model 4 Strength Related to the Number of Dilutions
Potency (C)	Strength Relative to Original Nondiluted Material or Tincture			
0	1	1	1	0
1	10^2	2	1.01	1
2	10^4	4	1.02	2
6	10^{12}	64	1.06	6
12	10^{24}	4,096	1.13	12
30	10^{60}	1.0×10^9	1.35	30
100	10^{200}	1.3×10^{30}	2.70	100
200	10^{400}	1.6×10^{60}	7.32	200
500	$10^{1,000}$	3.3×10^{150}	145	500
1,000	$10^{2,000}$	1.1×10^{301}	21,000	1,000
2,000	$10^{4,000}$	1.2×10^{602}	4.4×10^8	2,000
5,000	$10^{10,000}$	$1.4 \times 10^{1,505}$	4.0×10^{21}	5,000
10,000	$10^{20,000}$	$2.0 \times 10^{3,010}$	1.6×10^{43}	10,000
20,000	$10^{40,000}$	$4.0 \times 10^{6,020}$	2.7×10^{86}	20,000
50,000	$10^{100,000}$	$3.2 \times 10^{15,051}$	1.2×10^{216}	50,000
100,000	$10^{200,000}$	$1.0 \times 10^{30,103}$	1.4×10^{432}	100,000

Table 6.3. Remedy Strengths Under Various Assumptions

In Model 4, how might homeopaths compare the strength of a 20,000C to a 10,000C remedy? Twenty thousand is 10,000 more than 10,000, and it is also twice as big as 10,000. If homeopaths feel that a 20,000C remedy is 10,000 times as strong as a 10,000C remedy, that is a big jump; one might wonder if some patients might need something in between. If, on the other hand, homeopaths feel that the 20,000C remedy is only twice as strong as a 10,000C remedy, then it is curious that the first 10,000 stages of potentization increased remedy strength by about a factor of 10,000, and the next 10,000 stages only increased remedy strength by a factor of two.

Here is another curiosity. Some homeopaths advocate that patients should gradually increase the potency of their medication in a process homeopaths call plussing. For the first dose, the patient dissolves the remedy in a glass of water and then takes a small amount, perhaps a teaspoonful. For the next dose, the patient pours out all but a few drops or a teaspoonful from the glass, adds water, and stirs. This is then a slightly higher potency dose. The process can be repeated many times. If the initial remedy was a 200C, then the subsequent doses might represent 201C, 202C, 203C, and so on. It is curious that such small changes in potency are thought to be effective when homeopaths believe there is no need to stock remedies anywhere in between 200C and 1,000C. Apparently homeopaths believe the change in potency is much more important than the potency itself.

Homeopaths might say that this analysis is fundamentally flawed; different potencies represent qualitatively different remedies. Thus it makes no sense to compare the strengths of two different potencies quantitatively. Yet, if different potencies are qualitatively different remedies, then why does it not matter more which potency is used?

In practice, homeopaths are not inclined to view remedy potencies so quantitatively, perhaps because proposed mathematical models seem to make no sense. Either very large differences in remedy strength do not matter much, or the huge number of extra potentization stages needed to achieve the more potent remedies does not affect strength very much. Neither seems plausible. Although these four models do not exhaust all possibilities, most reasonably simple models will have similar problems. None of these models is consistent with homeopathic practice, and of course, any quantitative model suggests that the amount of a remedy taken should matter, a claim that many homeopaths deny. Therefore, homeopathy seems to *require* that there be no quantification of remedy strength.

DOSE SIZE: PHYSICAL FORM AND AMOUNT

The most common ingestible homeopathic remedies come in three primary forms: liquid, spherical sugar pellets, and tablets (larger nonspherical pills). Pellets, also called globules or pilules, come in many sizes (figure 6.1); the sizes are named as the length in millimeters of ten contiguous pellets in a line (that is, ten times the diameter of one pellet in mm). Numbers 10, 20, and 35 are common, but others are also used.

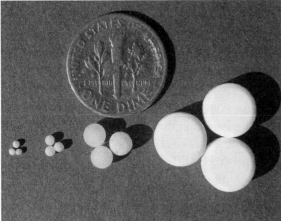

	#10: very small pellets, also called poppyseeds: diameter of 1 mm or a little over $\frac{1}{32}$ inch
	#20: small pellet diameter of 2 mm or a little over $\frac{1}{16}$ inch
	#35: regular pellets diameter of 3.5 mm or about $\frac{1}{8}$ inch
	#55: large pellets: diameter of 5.5 mm or between $\frac{1}{4}$ and $\frac{1}{8}$ inch (not shown)

Figure 6.1. #10, #20, and #35 pellets, and tablets.

In conventional medicine, the amount prescribed as a dose is critical, and there is usually an optimum dose. If the dose is ten times too small, it has no effect; if the dose is ten times too large, the result can be detrimental or even fatal. In addition, in conventional medicine there are multiple ways of getting the same dose. One 400 mg pill has the same effect as two 200 mg pills; the amount of medicine is what counts.

In homeopathy, typical suggestions for the quantities to be taken at one time are:

#10 and #20 pellets: five to fifteen, or a lidful
#35 and #55 pellets: one to five
Liquid: five to twenty-five drops (about 0.1 to 0.5 **mL**)[8]
Tablets: one

Despite these dose suggestions, the most startling fact is that many homeopaths say it does not matter how much remedy is taken at one time. This claim is so striking that a sampling of supporting quotations is appropriate.

Dana Ullman: "The number of homeopathic pills, globules, pellets, or drops to take per dose is generally not considered as vital to a therapeutic response as is the correct remedy, potency, and frequency of repetition."[9]

Richard Moskowitz: "The size of the dose, the actual number of granules or tablets ingested, is of negligible importance under most circumstances."[10]

Rajendra Upadhyay: "The size (number of globules) of a dose is also immaterial in prescribing."[11]

Miranda Castro: "If your child gets her hands on a bottle of pills and eats the entire first-aid kit in one glorious secret feast, do not panic. Your bank balance is the only thing that will suffer. A single dose at one time is a single dose, whether it is one pill or one bottle of pills—for example, eating a full bottle of Chamomilla 6 tablets would have the same effect as taking one single pill."[12]

More evidence that the amount taken does not matter is the internal inconsistency in the typical recommended doses of pellets versus liquid. If five drops of liquid remedy is equivalent to one #35 pellet, this presents an apparent inconsistency of a factor of two hundred, since five drops is enough to medicate about two hundred pellets.[13]

The remedy is supposed to stimulate the body to heal itself. Yet if this stimulation is due to something in the remedies, whether material or immaterial, it would seem that a two hundred-fold overdose due either to consuming a whole bottle of two hundred pellets or to taking five drops instead of one pellet might have a different effect. Some homeopaths claim that dose matters when treating chronic cases or especially sensitive patients, but few feel it is critical for most acute cases.

Even though many homeopaths believe that the number of pills taken does not matter,[14] most homeopaths nevertheless recommend particular numbers of pills or drops. The following may be some of the reasons. (1) The dose amounts may be decided upon partly for convenience—the smallest pills are too small to count easily, so a lidful is suggested; the larger pills and the tablets can easily be handled singly and counted, so a particular small number is specified; (2) It is too difficult to convince the public that dose does not matter; (3) Many homeopaths also find the dose-doesn't-matter concept uncomfortable and easily slip back into the conventional medicine notion that the amount matters. (4) For over-the-counter remedies there is one more and a rather mundane reason for specifying a particular dose—the Food and Drug Administration requires dose recommendations be on the bottle.

DOSE FREQUENCY AND NUMBER OF REPETITIONS

For chronic ailments, the interval between doses is usually relatively long, typically from a month to more than a year. For acute ailments, the time between doses may be minutes, hours, or days. The number of times the remedy is taken varies from only once to a few; if no improvement is seen

after about six doses, most homeopaths assume that the remedy is wrong
and consider changing it.

In almost all cases, homeopaths believe that the number of doses taken
should be as few as possible. The overriding principle is to stop the remedy
when there is improvement; the homeopathic reason is so that the improvement can continue without interference. One form of claimed interference
is an **inadvertent proving**: If a remedy is taken too many times, the patient
may develop the symptoms that the remedy is intended to cure.

Nonetheless, a few homeopaths advocate continuing to take the
remedy despite improvement. In some cases they recommend taking a
remedy every thirty seconds for up to twenty minutes,[15] and in other cases
they recommend dosing ten times a day and continuing with the same set
of remedies for a year or more.[16] Thus, different homeopaths claim that different and contradictory approaches are effective.

MINIMUM DOSE

One of Hahnemann's fundamental principles was the use of the minimum dose.
Probably he formulated this principle to minimize side effects from ingesting
too much of toxic remedies such as mercury, arsenic, and belladonna; that is,
he wanted to minimize the real chemical dose. Now that very few remedies are
used in potencies that could conceivably have any chemically based side
effects, it is not clear how to interpret Hahnemann's minimum dose dictum.
Castro, Jonas and Jacobs, and Panos and Heimlich all appear to associate minimum dose with high dilution and hence high potency.[17] Herscu seems to
believe just the opposite—that minimum dose means using the least potent
remedy.[18] Moskowitz and Cummings[19] believe that minimum dose means
taking the remedy the smallest number of times and having longer intervals
between repetitions. De Schepper believes that Hahnemann meant the smallest
number of pellets.[20] Sollar's interpretation is that minimum dose means taking
only one remedy at a time.[21] It is interesting that there are such blatantly contradictory views on one of the most fundamental principles of homeopathy.

STORING THE REMEDY

A number of homeopaths claim that, if properly stored, homeopathic remedies can remain active for at least a century or two if not indefinitely.[22]

However, improper storage conditions are claimed to deactivate the remedies. These conditions include the following:

- Temperature above 100 degrees Fahrenheit.[23] Some homeopaths say that up to 130 degrees is safe.[24]
- High humidity.
- Long-term exposure to direct sunlight or other bright light.
- Storage in an environment with certain strong smells, including solvents, paints, camphor, perfumes, nail polish or its remover, mothballs, mint, and menthol. Storing homeopathic remedies with typical personal items such as ointments and mouthwashes is not advised.
- Exposure to excessive microwaves, x-rays, steady electric and magnetic fields, and low-frequency electromagnetic radiation, including 60 Hertz radiation, as from electric blankets, electric motors, and house wiring.
- Hard knocks,[25] such as a remedy bottle falling and landing on an uncarpeted floor.
- Transferring the remedy from its original container to a different bottle.
- Leaving the cap loose or off for more than the time needed to dispense the remedy.
- Having more than one bottle open at a time: "Cross-potentization may result if this precaution is not observed."[26]

Thinking about these precautions raises some questions:

- Why would storing the bottle in the presence of high humidity or vapors matter if the bottles are sealed?
- The natural environment contains electric fields, magnetic fields, x-rays, and microwaves. If the deactivating effects of these influences on remedies are cumulative, then it may be surprising that any remedies as much as one hundred years old are still active.
- Similarly, why would direct sunlight for a short time be any worse than indirect sunlight or indoor lighting for a long time, given that the same number of photons might have hit the remedy? Photographic film can be exposed either with intense light for a short time or by dim light over a long time.
- It is curious that storage above 100° F is thought to deactivate remedies, given that the official guidelines for remedy preparation permit drying of the pellets and tablets at temperatures somewhat above 100° F.[27]

It is difficult to find definitive answers in homeopathy. Despite the published claims of some homeopaths who believe that 100° F will ruin remedies, others say there are no effects until around 200° F. Some believe that airport x-ray machines deactivate remedies, but others who travel by air "as much as once or twice per week . . . report that medicines are still effective."[28]

The evidence for these claimed storage effects is probably anecdotal. In the past, practitioners naturally looked for explanations when a patient did not get better after taking the remedy. In a few cases, they realized that the remedy had been left in sunlight or near a hot stove, or subjected to x-rays at an airport. They jumped to the conclusion that strong light (or high temperatures or x-rays) deactivated remedies, and this belief became their internal reality. Such erroneous leaps are common, but correlation is not cause: B preceding A does not necessarily mean that B caused A. There are many other possible reasons for patients not responding to homeopathic remedies. Establishing the external reality of remedy deactivation requires either a lab test (which at present does not exist) for the remedy's active ingredient or determining whether a remedy that is known to heal unambiguously almost every time (no such remedy has yet been found) does not work after it has been exposed to claimed deactivating agents.

TAKING THE REMEDY

There are many ways to take a homeopathic remedy. In a recent study at the Glasgow Homeopathic Hospital, the doctors gave thirteen different sets of instructions for how to take the same remedy.[29] The following procedures are common; homeopaths claim that failure to follow any part of the process may result in the remedy having no effect:

- Remedies should be taken without anyone touching them. The pill(s) can be tipped out into the lid of the bottle and from there into the patient's mouth. Second best is to allow the patient, but no one else, to touch the pills.
- The pills should not be chewed; they should just dissolve in the mouth, under the tongue according to some homeopaths.
- Liquid remedies should not be swallowed right away but should be left in the mouth for a few seconds.
- If a pill falls out of the bottle onto the floor, a table, or other furniture, it should be discarded.

- Most homeopaths advise against eating or drinking anything within fifteen to thirty minutes before and after taking a remedy.
- Remedies should not be administered outdoors or near windows if that would result in their exposure to direct sunlight, even if the exposure is only for a few seconds.

Another technique is to dissolve the pill in water and then drink some or all of the solution. The patient must be careful to use a very clean container and stirrer.

Some homeopaths use much more elaborate methods. An example is Dr. A. U. Ramakrishnan's technique for helping cancer patients:

> Put three pills (pellets) in eleven spoons of water. Take one spoonful every fifteen minutes with a gentle shake or stir in between, for ten spoonfuls each day; save the last spoonful to carry over for the next day. Start the next day's dose with that last spoonful, adding ten more spoonfuls of water and then dosing as before. After one week, discard the last spoonful and switch to the nosode, dosing it the same way. After a week of the nosode, go back to the first remedy, beginning again with the initial potency and plussing as before.[30]

LM remedies have their own distinctive protocol as specified by Hahnemann and interpreted more succinctly by De Schepper:

> The patient takes one poppyseed pellet and places it in a 4 oz. (100 mL approximately) standard pharmacy bottle, then fills the bottle to the base of the neck with purified water and adds fifteen drops of ethanol. The patient succusses the bottle each day before taking a dose, giving the bottle a hard blow against the palm of his hand or a leather-bound book. The number of succussions is adjusted to the sensitivity level of the patient, typically from two to eight times. Then the patient pours one teaspoon from the remedy bottle into a cup with 4 oz. (100 mL) of purified water, stirs well, and takes one teaspoon (5 mL) as the daily dose. The patient begins with LM1, typically for three weeks then moves on to LM2, then LM3; most chronic cases are cured before the patient reaches LM10. This is the standard way of administering LMs for non-sensitive patients. Hypersensitive patients need adjustment of the dose.[31]

Since the bottle is shaken daily, homeopaths believe that the potency increases slightly each day, enhancing the healing process.

What are the reasons for not touching the remedy? Most homeopathy books give no reasons, but Steven Kayne states: "Solid dose forms are not handled, so as to minimize the possibility of bacterial or chemical contamination."[32] However, such conventional contamination seems unlikely to be critical since it is everywhere, and other homeopathic medication methods involve using glasses and spoons that have been handled without such precautions. In addition, no similar precautions are thought to be necessary for virtually all other types of oral medication. We put things in our mouths all the time that we have touched with our hands—primarily food—and rarely suffer ill effects.

Another theory for why the remedy should not be handled is that touching the pill rubs off some of the active ingredient. This seems inconsequential given that only a tiny fraction of the pill's mass will be lost, and given homeopathy's disregard for the size of the dose anyway. It is also curious that no one seems to be concerned that homeopathic ointments are of course touched by the patient or by a caregiver. Why would touching a pill deactivate the pill if applying an ointment does not deactivate the ointment?

A strictly homeopathic reason for not handling remedies could be that hands might have a strong odor (e.g., from soap, lotion, candy, or gasoline), and strong odors are believed to "antidote" the remedy. If odors do matter, then one only need sniff one's hands. If there is no strong odor, handling the remedy should be no problem.

Another homeopathic reason why people other than the patient should not touch the remedy is that just touching a remedy can be equivalent to taking it. Dana Ullman says: "As for being affected by a homeopathic medicine simply by touching it, there are some cases of this happening, though it is rarely a problem because the person touching the remedy is most often the person taking it."[33] Since the remedy was prescribed only for the patient, anyone else touching it might suffer from an inadvertent proving.

Some conventional drugs, for example nitroglycerine, can be absorbed just by skin contact, whereas others, such as insulin, cannot. Therefore, without knowing what the active ingredient in homeopathic remedies is, one cannot predict whether skin absorption is likely.

What is the evidence behind all of these remedy-taking precautions? Deactivation due to touching or dropping the remedy is one possible explanation, but there are many others. The only way to know that the touching was the actual cause is through careful testing. Again, such testing requires measurement of active ingredients or consistently curative remedies, neither of which is currently available.

What is the evidence for the assertion that when someone other than the patient touches the remedy, the remedy acts on that person? Occasionally someone who touches a remedy may get the same symptoms as if they took the remedy. The question is the cause of the symptoms. One mechanism is just chance. Another is the contagiousness of some diseases: Occasionally a caregiver contracts the patient's disease, and this unfortunate event would resemble an inadvertent proving.

Finally, it seems contradictory that homeopaths do not object to caregivers using their fingers to get remedies into the mouths of unconscious patients and babies. Homeopathy's rules seem to bend when it is inconvenient or impossible to follow them.

DOES THE INTAKE METHOD MATTER?

Homeopaths seem to assume that how medications contact one's body does not affect their action. The same remedy is sometimes available in different forms, such as oral tablets or drops, ointments or injections. They are all presumed to be effective even though virtually all provings are oral.

Outside of homeopathy, intake mode is often critical. Sucrose is effective taken orally or intravenously; topically it has no effect, and if sucrose is injected into muscle or skin, it causes the tissue to rot and die. Oxygen needs to be supplied to the lungs, not to the stomach or skin. Penicillin and aspirin do not work when applied topically.

Homeopathic remedies are supposed to work by stimulating the vital force, but the vital force has no specific location in the body; it is not even material. Then why would it be more beneficial to apply a remedy locally where there are symptoms, as in ointments and eye drops or nasal sprays? The vital force does not live in a skin rash. If locally applied ointments are effective, perhaps the benefit is due to physical effects of its application (rubbing) or to biochemical effects of the ointment base.

CONCLUSION

If potency is not critical; if the amount of remedy taken often does not matter; if stopping the remedy or continuing to take it both work; and if oral, topical, and injectable forms of the same remedy all work, one might wonder if homeopathic cures are effective for reasons other than the remedies.

NOTES

1. Dana Ullman, *The Consumer's Guide to Homeopathy* (New York: G. P. Putnam's Sons, 1995), p. 92.

2. Will Taylor, "Many Strategies of Prescribing," *Homeopathy Today* 22, no. 2 (2002): 32–33.

3. Elizabeth Wright-Hubbard, *A Brief Study Course in Homeopathy* (St. Louis: Formur, Inc., 1997), p. 46.

4. Jay Yasgur, *Homeopathic Dictionary* (Greenville, Penn.: Van Hoy Publishers, 1998), p. 6.

5. James Stephenson, "A Review of Investigations into the Action of Substances in Solutions Greater Than 1×10^{-24} (Microdilutions)," *Journal of the American Institute of Homeopathy* 48, no. 11 (1995): 79–94.

6. Julie Bernard, *Potency in Homeopathic Prescribing* (Mill Valley, Calif.: self-published, 1999), p. 108.

7. Registered name of Heel, Inc.

8. For water dispensed from a typical dropper, twenty drops is about 1 mL. Liquid homeopathic remedies are typically 20 percent alcohol, and for this water/alcohol mixture, drop size is significantly smaller than for pure water—roughly twice as many drops per mL.

9. Ullman, p. 95.

10. Richard Moskowitz, *Resonance: The Homeopathic Point of View* (http://www.Xlibris.com, Xlibris Corporation, 2000), p. 36.

11. Rajendra Upadhyay, letter to the editor, *Homeopathy* (formerly the *British Homeopathic Journal*) 91, no. 4 (2002): 268.

12. Miranda Castro, *The Complete Book of Homeopathy* (New York: St. Martin's Press, 1990), p. 25.

13. The specific HPUS instructions are as follows: "The globules are medicated by placing them in a vial and adding the liquid drug attenuation in the proportion not less than 1 percent, volume by weight (i.e., one (1) drop for 2 g or 1 dram), and shaking to obtain a uniform medication." Two grams of #35 pellets is about forty-four pellets.

The notion that the amount taken does not matter stands in contrast to the quantitative care with which the remedies are manufactured. The HPUS specifications effectively require on the order of 1 percent precision (no more than 1 percent error). Yet taking five drops of liquid remedy instead of one regular pellet delivers about 20,000 percent more medicine.

14. In contrast to the conventional homeopathic wisdom that the amount does not matter, the makers of some combination remedies apparently think that at least the *relative* amount of each remedy *does* matter because they specify different amounts of each remedy.

Ingredients in Atropinum Compositum	
(a Heel-brand combination remedy for colic)	
Ingredient	**Percentage by Volume**
Atropinum sulphuricum 4X	99.9
Bryonia alba 0	0.02
Berberis vulgaris 0	0.01
Pareira brava 0	0.01
Colocynthis 0	0.01
Veratrum album 0	0.01
Cuprum aceticum 2X	0.01
Arsenicum album 4X	0.01
Baptisia tinctoria 0	0.003
Chelidonium majus 0	0.003
Cantharus 5X	0.001
Medorrhinum 10X	0.001
Thuja occidentalis 0	0.0003
Clematis erecta 0	0.0003
Benzoicum acidum 2X	0.0001
Argentum nitricum 1X	0.00001

15. Isaac Chan, "Rapid Dose (R.D.) Techniques: Treating a Case of Life-Threatening Hydrothorax," *Simillimum* 13, no. 3 (2000): 66–85.

16. A. U. Ramakrishnan and Catherine R. Coulter, *A Homeopathic Approach to Cancer* (St. Louis: Quality Medical Publishing, 2001), p. 15.

17. Castro, p. 12; Wayne Jonas and Jennifer Jacobs, *Healing with Homeopathy: The Doctors' Guide* (New York: Warner Books, 1996), p. 17; and Maesimund Panos and Jane Heimlich, *Homeopathic Medicine at Home* (Los Angeles: J. P. Tarcher, 1980), p. 42.

18. Paul Herscu, *Provings Volume, with a Proving of Alcoholus* (Amherst, Mass.: New England School of Homeopathy Press, 2002), p. 96.

19. Moskowitz, p. 35; Stephen Cummings with Dana Ullman, *Everybody's Guide to Homeopathic Medicines* (New York: Jeremy P. Tarcher/Putnam, 1997), p. 9.

20. Luc De Schepper, *Hahnemann Revisited* (Santa Fe: Full of Life Publishing, 2001), p. 85.

21. David Sollars, *The Complete Idiot's Guide to Homeopathy* (Indianapolis: Alpha Books, 2002), p. 62.

22. Castro, p. 25; Steven Kayne, *Homeopathic Pharmacy* (New York: Churchill Livingston, 1997), p. 58; Panos and Heimlich, p. 43; Cummings, p. 35.

23. Ullman, p. 151.

24. "A Guide for Taking Homeopathic Remedies" [online], http://www.homeopathyworks.com/guide.htm [May 18, 2002].

25. Peter Morrell, "Reply to Adams and FitzGerald," *British Medical Journal* [online], http://bmj.com/cgi/eletters/321/7259/471#9872 [Nov. 29, 2002].

26. Cummings, p. 35.

27. *The Homeopathic Pharmacopoeia of the United States, Abstracts: 2001* (HPUS) (Washington, D.C.: Homoeopathic Pharmacopoeia Convention of the United States, 2001), p. 44.

28. "Frequently Asked Questions," *Homeopathy Today* 21, no. 11 (2001): 37.

29. Steven Kayne, "A Study of Remedies Prescribed at Glasgow Homeopathic Hospital," *British Homeopathic Journal* 87, no. 4 (1998): 190–94.

30. A. U. Ramakrishnan, "Homeopathy in Breast Cancer: A Bright Outlook," *Journal of the American Institute of Homeopathy* 93, no. 1 (2000): 41.

31. Luc De Schepper, "LM Potencies: One of the Hidden Treasures of the Sixth Edition of the *Organon*," *British Homeopathic Journal* 88 (1999): 128–34.

32. Kayne, *Homeopathic Pharmacy*, p. 74.

33. Ullman, p. 150.

7. Following the Patient's Progress

T he patient has now taken the remedy. What happens next? Sometimes the patient gets better, sometimes worse, and sometimes he or she stays the same. Sometimes the original symptoms get worse, and sometimes new symptoms arise. Sometimes the patient gets worse physically but improves mentally or emotionally, and sometimes the reverse happens. Sometimes the worsening lasts only hours or days, and sometimes it lasts weeks or months. Sometimes a deterioration of the patient's condition is followed by an improvement; sometimes improvement is followed by a relapse.

All of these responses can follow any health care intervention; patients do not always just improve. Reasons can include the natural vicissitudes of most ailments, side effects of the treatment, misdiagnosis of the problem and consequently wrong intervention, new unrelated problems, different sensitivities of patients to particular treatments, and health problems so advanced and severe that no intervention can save the patient.

However, homeopathy has a number of uniquely homeopathic reasons for the patients' not getting completely well after taking a remedy. Many of these explanations seem plausible, but are they valid? What kind of observations would it take to prove them valid? Or are they essentially just excuses, however plausible they may sound, to justify the fact that patients do not always get better? This chapter takes a critical look at homeopathic responses to the patient's progress.

AGGRAVATION

Homeopaths are encouraged when they see a patient's symptoms get worse after taking a remedy. Maesimund Panos and Jane Heimlich describe the case of Mr. Smith, who had been suffering from stomachaches:

> On Mr. Smith's return visit, I give him a single high potency dose of Nux vomica and ask that he report any changes. . . . Two days later, Mr. Smith's wife calls. Her husband came home from work last evening complaining of a terrible stomachache. . . . I reassure her that his temporary upset is a normal response. . . . Mr. Smith's response illustrates the classic homeopathic "aggravation," a sign that the remedy is stimulating the patient's defense mechanism. The sick person is always ultra sensitive to his similar remedy. Just as a tuning fork responds by resonating to the properly struck note, so the individual given the similar medicine responds with an increase of all symptoms. I am always happy to have a patient report an aggravation, as this usually shows that the remedy was the right one. An aggravation generally lasts a day or two and is followed by improvement.[1]

Why should a homeopathic remedy make the symptoms worse? Undesirable side effects can certainly result from treatments of any sort, but very few other types of interventions cause the primary symptoms to worsen as a helpful and desirable part of the cure; fevers don't increase, tumors don't grow, headaches don't worsen, bacterial counts don't increase because of nonhomeopathic treatments directed at the specific complaint. Yes, homeopathy is different, which is why it is so intriguing, but also why it should receive more scrutiny.

George Vithoulkas offers a homeopathic explanation for aggravations:

> The homeopathic aggravation can be considered as a way in which the organism is "encouraged" by the indicated medicine to "confess," to bring to light deep-seated troubles or evil tendencies that were oppressing it before. To be completely free, an organism must be fully expressive and creative in the context of its immediate reality. When its expression is inhibited, suppressed, rendered secret, or obstructed, then we have an ill individual. . . . The remedy then produces a stimulation of

the defense mechanism, which creates for a time a heightened exacerbation of the symptoms which are the only manifestation of its action visible to our perception.[2]

At best this is only a metaphor: it certainly is not a testable theory.

How common are aggravations? Low estimates are that about 10 to 20 percent of patients feel worse initially.[3] Vithoulkas and his colleagues claim that about 70 percent of patients feel worse initially,[4] when Vithoulkas sees a cure without an aggravation, one of his explanations for this lack of aggravation is that the "case was already severely aggravated at the outset."[5] In the case of severe chronic headaches, some homeopaths, including Vithoulkas, even *guarantee* that the patient will get worse before getting better.[6]

How does the homeopath know at the time whether a worsening of symptoms is an aggravation or the patient's getting worse because the remedy was not effective? There is no way to tell. If the patient ultimately gets well, then the homeopath will declare that the worsening was a good sign. If the patient does not get well, the homeopath may claim that the remedy was wrong or was antidoted or provide some other reasons. Hindsight is required.

Homeopaths interpret aggravations as evidence that healing is taking place. However, there are other more mundane explanations. The natural vicissitudes of many ailments guarantee that some patients will feel worse, whether or not they take a remedy. The power of suggestion may explain some aggravations: patients are told the remedy may make their symptoms get worse. A lifestyle change recommended by the homeopath can even produce an intensification of symptoms and then a cure, mimicking a homeopathic aggravation. For instance, if a headache sufferer is a heavy coffee drinker, then stopping the caffeine intake, which homeopaths recommend, often produces a few intense headaches before they wane; this effect appears to be aggravation followed by cure but also happens without a homeopathic remedy.

Is it actually true that a worsening of symptoms is a good sign? Statistically, the "good sign" aspect will often *appear* to be true since most patients naturally get better after getting worse. This effect, sometimes called **regression to the mean** (see chapter 8), is only the statistical illusion of healing. If the worsening of symptoms were *really* a good sign, then patients who initially get worse should ultimately be more likely to get well, get well faster, or stay well longer, or have less intense symptoms than patients who just get well without getting worse first.

There appears to be little if any quality evidence for homeopathic aggravations—that aggravations are *caused* by remedies and/or that, when they occur, the patient does get better in the future. In a recent (2003) systematic review of homeopathic aggravations in clinical trials, S. Grabia and Edzard Ernst concluded that "this systematic review does not provide clear evidence that the phenomena of homeopathic aggravation exists."[7]

ANTIDOTING DUE TO PATIENT ACTIONS

Homeopaths claim that remedies can be deactivated by exposure to certain environmental factors, as explained in the previous chapter. Homeopaths also claim that a good, active remedy, properly taken, may be prevented from helping a patient by certain patient actions. Thus, any of the following can ostensibly cause the correct remedy to fail:

- The patient drank coffee (some homeopaths also impugn decaffeinated coffee or even just coffee flavor).
- The patient drank tea or citrus juice.
- The patient consumed alcohol or chocolate.
- The patient ate spicy foods, including onion, garlic, hot peppers, or cayenne spice.
- The patient ate highly processed or "chemicalized" foods.[8]
- The patient took high doses of vitamins.[9]
- The patient smoked.
- The patient took a mineral bath.[10]
- The patient indulged in recreational drugs (beyond caffeine, alcohol, and nicotine).
- The patient did not exercise adequately.
- The patient's diet was not healthful.
- The patient used a cellular phone.
- The patient did not get enough sleep.
- The patient did not deal with stress.
- The patient was exposed to certain strong odors, such as those from perfume; certain cough lozenges, especially those containing menthol; certain deep heat ointments, especially those containing camphor; certain essential oils such as rosemary, eucalyptus, and pennyroyal[11]; ammonia; hair permanents; moth balls; cleaning agents; or paint and paint thinner. Homeopaths do not agree on the details and suggest that patients may have different susceptibilities to odors.

- The patient was exposed to excessive electromagnetic fields, such as from sleeping under an electric blanket or using a hair dryer.
- Pesticides were used at or near the patient's home or place of work.
- The patient was exposed to an animal and had an allergic reaction.
- An emotional shock, such as some bad news, blocked the cure.

DOES COFFEE ANTIDOTE HOMEOPATHIC REMEDIES?

American homeopath Timothy Dooley says, "Coffee is not a food; it is not nutritive. Its effects are medicinal and drug-like. . . . The use of coffee often interferes with remedies."[12] Another American homeopath, David Sollars, argues, "In Europe, where homeopathy has flourished for two centuries, they drink very strong coffee and still experience improvement from remedies."[13] As is so often the case, homeopaths disagree with one another.

Some homeopaths also believe that each remedy has its own specific food taboos. For instance, it is considered important for a patient being treated with Kali carbonicum to avoid meat, vegetables, milk, pancakes, black bread, cold drinks, fats, and ice, as well as coffee,[14] whereas if the remedy is Cimicifuga racemosa, only liquors and sour foods are of concern.[15]

Similarly, almost any nonhomeopathic health care intervention can ostensibly antidote the action of a homeopathic remedy:

- An **allopathic (conventional) medicine**, such as strong painkillers, antibiotics, sedatives, or tranquillizers suppressed the patient's defenses.[16]
- The patient had an MRI (magnetic resonance image).
- Ultrasound was used on the patient.[17]
- A visit to the dentist blocked the cure.[18]
- The patient had local or general anesthesia.[19]
- Other alternative health care practices, such as acupuncture, chiropractic, reiki, osteopathy, hypnosis, yoga, polarity therapy, craniosacral manipulation, Bach flower remedies, or herbs antidoted, exaggerated, or confused the homeopathic remedy.[20]

Some homeopaths believe that although X and C remedies are susceptible to all these antidoting problems, LM remedies are not, or at least are much less so.[21] Apparently, the slight differences in how remedies are diluted and how many times they are succussed can have profound effects on their properties.

Is all this true? No doubt in some cases when any of the above events occurred, the patient did not improve after homeopathic treatment, but such instances do not necessarily indicate a causal relationship. There are many other reasons why a patient might not respond. Again, if homeopathic remedies almost always worked, then testing the effects of tranquilizers or acupuncture on their effectiveness would be relatively easy. But they don't, so it isn't.

Evidence that is convincing for many homeopaths is exemplified by the following statement by Robert Ullman and Judyth Reichenberg-Ullman: "Acupuncture and therapeutic ultrasound have been known to disturb homeopathic treatment in some cases, although both may also have significant therapeutic value."[22] This statement probably means that at least one patient who failed to improve after taking a homeopathic remedy was also being treated with acupuncture or ultrasound. Only one of the many possible explanations for why the patient did not improve is that acupuncture and ultrasound disturbed the homeopathic remedies. Researcher Wayne Jonas and homeopath Jennifer Jacobs acknowledge: "No scientific study has been conducted to verify [antidoting]."[23]

Researcher Harald Walach also has doubts about the phenomenon of antidoting:

> The homeopathic debate about antidoting is as fascinating as a Harry Potter saga, and as fictitious. Let us keep in mind how the antidoting debate started: Hahnemann sought a scapegoat for missing homeopathic effects, where he expected them. His scapegoats were coffee, strong spices, alcohol, and a lot of other stuff. Interestingly enough, tobacco is missing from [his] list, probably because Hahnemann was a pipe smoker."[24]

It would be extremely difficult for homeopathic patients to follow all the antidoting admonitions. It seems unlikely that homeopathy could have its claimed success if half of these actions reliably antidoted the remedies. Furthermore, if spicy food were an antidote, then homeopathy could not enjoy its very strong following in India and many other parts of the world. The evidence suggests that all these claimed antidotes are just excuses.

INADVERTENT PROVINGS

If the remedy is wrong, the patient may be made worse, according to homeopaths. When any remedy is given to a healthy or ill person, a proving reaction can result: The person gets some of the symptoms that the remedy is believed capable of curing. If the patient is especially sensitive, a single dose can induce the symptoms.

Some homeopaths believe that combination remedies are more likely to cause inadvertent provings than single remedies since either all or all but one of the components of the mixture are not the simillimum. Steven Kayne comments: "My colleague Dr. Stuart Semple of Edinburgh tells me that in his experience unnecessary components can give violent aggravations (often when least needed)."[25]

The evidence for inadvertent provings, like that for antidoting, is probably only anecdotal. Homeopaths undoubtedly observe some patients getting worse, sometimes with new symptoms that belong to the remedy. However, these observations are insufficient to establish a cause/effect relationship.

HERING'S LAWS

A nineteenth-century physician named Constantine Hering compiled some homeopathic theories on how symptoms should evolve after taking the correct remedy, or how a practitioner can tell if the patient is healing properly. These theories have come to be known as **Hering's Laws** even though they were never so labeled during his lifetime.

If patients simply got better after homeopathic treatment, there would be no need for these laws. But since they do not, homeopaths believe that it is a good sign if the patient's symptoms evolve as described by Hering's Laws despite the fact that the symptoms are not just going away.

Some authors divide Hering's ideas into three laws and others into four; the four-law version is presented here, with names supplied for convenience in referencing them. Two versions of each law are presented: one that concerns a patient with multiple symptoms and the order in which the symptoms disappear and another that concerns new symptoms that may arise during the healing process.

When the patient has multiple symptoms, it is considered a sign that the remedy is working if the symptoms disappear according to one of the following guidelines:

Hering's most-important-first law: In order from more important to less important. Since the brain is more important than the skin, if a patient was originally suffering from headaches and skin rashes, the headaches should improve first.

Hering's inside-out law: In order from inside the body to outside. If the symptoms include digestive problems and skin rash, the digestive problem should be relieved before the skin rash.

Hering's top-down law: In order from head downward to toes. If the original symptoms include sinus problems and sore ankles, the sinus problems should clear up first.

If the patient develops new symptoms while the old symptoms are waning, the remedy is working if either of the following conditions is met:

Hering's most-important-first, inside-out, and top-down laws: As the old symptoms are waning, the basic malady moves to less important organs, to more exterior parts of the body, or to lower parts of the body. As mental or emotional symptoms are improving, the appearance of joint, muscle, tendon, or skin problems is a good sign.

Hering's reverse-order law: The new symptoms are from old ailments the patient had in the past, and they arise and wane in reverse order of their original incidence.

Hering's reverse-order law is more complex than the others. Many homeopaths believe that if old ailments were not cured homeopathically, they were not really cured; they were suppressed. When a patient finally experiences a first homeopathic cure for a specific ailment, then this same homeopathic remedy can ostensibly cure all the previous ailments as well. This curing process is revealed by the reappearance of all the old ailments' symptoms in the reverse order in which the patient had them. The first old symptom to arise will be from the most recent ailment; the last will be from a very early childhood disease. Thus a patient receiving a homeopathic remedy for allergies may temporarily get eczema if years ago the patient had eczema that was suppressed with steroid ointments. (Some homeopaths suspect that the patient may even develop symptoms from diseases he or she never had but that their parents or grandparents had.)[26]

Hering's Laws are not as impressive as they may sound. They are too loosely stated to be readily testable and the evolution of symptoms may have plausible nonhomeopathic causes. The following paragraphs illustrate these flaws.

1. Testing the most-important-first law requires an unambiguous definition of *most important*. Ambiguity is inevitable. Jonas and Jacobs state:

   > The most important of these principles is that when a person is healing
   > properly, he or she will get better first in areas that are the most crucial to
   > his or her ability to function. For example, if a person with allergies also
   > has mental confusion and severe fatigue, a positive response to a homeo-
   > pathic remedy might be an improvement in the confusion and fatigue
   > before there is any change in the allergies. . . . On the other hand, if the
   > allergy symptoms are so severe as to limit the person's functioning more
   > than fatigue, one would expect that the allergies would improve to a
   > greater extent and before (or simultaneously with) the fatigue."[27]

   It is clearly a matter of judgment as to which symptom is most debilitating. There is also some ambiguity in deciding how much improvement
   in a symptom is sufficient to declare that it improved.

2. There is at least one explanation other than Hering's Laws for why a
   patient's mental outlook might improve before the physical symptoms
   do. Patients are often scared and confused about their ailments before
   seeking professional help. The biggest fear, that the ailment may be
   permanent or fatal, is depressing and debilitating. A consultation with
   any health practitioner usually allays such fears. The patient's mental
   outlook is improved by the office visit. However, the homeopath will
   probably attribute the increased confidence to the remedy itself and
   point out that this is improvement is in accordance with Hering's Laws.

3. The most debilitating symptom may improve first due to regression to
   the mean (see chapter 8). The most severe symptom is more likely than
   others to be near its maximum intensity and hence is more likely to get
   better if there is some random variability in symptom intensity.

4. Hering's Laws can conflict with one another. Should the excruciatingly
   painful foot problem be alleviated first, before the mild headaches,
   even though this would be healing from the bottom up instead of top
   down? Homeopaths say yes. When the laws conflict, they consider the
   whole person. The patient is thought to be on the right track as long as
   he or she "experiences an overall increase in health and freedom."[28]

5. Hering's reverse-order law is especially difficult to verify, partly because

the law itself needs clarification. Does it *always* happen that the first use of homeopathy brings back old symptoms from previous ailments?

- Do *all* old symptoms come back, or just some?
- Do the symptoms come back in *precise* reverse order?

Even if this law were clear, there would be significant hurdles in its verification:

- To identify all past ailments, does a practitioner rely on patient memory? This tactic is unreliable both for completeness and for relative timing. It is also difficult to obtain all medical records if a patient has had more than one primary care physician. Even medical records are not complete because professional help is not sought for every ailment. These difficulties make it unlikely that homeopaths have carefully tested Hering's fourth law to establish its external reality.
- Do old symptoms sometimes recur even though a homeopathic remedy was used and apparently cured them? Was the illness only suppressed (see the following section), perhaps because the remedy was not quite the simillimum, or not sufficiently potent? If so, a patient cannot know in advance which prior ailments should resurface, in which case the law cannot be tested.
- New symptoms can occur that have nothing to do with past ailments, perhaps caused by the patient contracting a new ailment during the cure. The difficulty of determining whether an additional symptom is due to a new condition or is a recurrence of an old problem complicates testing Hering's reverse-order law.

Hering's Laws are difficult to test in a rigorous fashion, and it appears that no such testing has been done. Nonetheless, Hering's Laws can seem valid because the evolution of the symptoms can often be made to fit them. This is not difficult because of the vagueness of the laws and the latitude taken in interpreting them. If retrospective fitting is the reality, the laws are useless for contemporaneously assessing the healing process; they merely provide the illusion or internal reality of order and reason.

Despite the wide latitude in interpreting Hering's Laws, occasionally a case may not fit the expected pattern. But for homeopaths, such an exception does not invalidate the laws. If a patient's progress does not fit, homeopaths believe that the remedy or dosing was wrong;[29] the laws only describe what happens in a *successful* cure. If a case does not fit, it is not counted, adding to the internal reality of the laws.

A few prominent homeopaths recognize the weaknesses in Hering's Laws. Dana Ullman appropriately called them "Hering's Guidelines" rather than laws.[30] Dr. André Saine said that neither he nor any other homeopath he has asked has confirmed Hering's Laws.[31]

SAFETY AND SIDE EFFECTS

Most people believe that homeopathic remedies are completely safe. Many books, remedy labels, brochures, and advertisements also assure safety, with phrases such as "all natural," "safe," "effective," and "no side effects." Are they really harmless?

The practice of homeopathy raises safety issues from two perspectives: conventional medicine and homeopathy itself. From the standpoint of conventional medicine, there are three types of risks from homeopathic care.

(1) The most serious risk is delayed effective medical treatment. It is essential that homeopaths, as well as all other health practitioners, realize the limitations of their practices and that they correctly diagnose life-threatening medical problems and send such patients to appropriate specialists. (2) Another risk can arise if homeopaths urge their patients to decrease or stop prescribed conventional medications. The physician who prescribed the medications should always be consulted. (3) Yet another medical risk of homeopathy is substituting homeopathic remedies for vaccinations, as discussed in chapter 12.

The *homeopathic* risks of homeopathy are not as well known to the public. While most of the public believe that homeopathy is free of side effects, the following quotations from respected homeopaths indicate otherwise:

Vithoulkas: "If it [the remedy] is originally a poisonous substance and it closely matches the resonant frequency of an oversensitive patient, a lower potency can produce a severe and dangerous aggravation."[32]

Ullman and Reichberg-Ullman: "Homeopathic pharmacies sometimes restrict the sale of high-potency remedies to practitioners only, as their safe use requires adequate training."[33]

Homeopaths state that symptoms can get worse or new symptoms can appear in response to taking a remedy, due to aggravations and

healing crises as described by Hering's Laws. The patient suffers, but homeopaths do not consider these discomforts to be side effects because they believe these reactions to be part of, or a direct indication of, the healing process. Thus it seems that homeopaths have eliminated side effects by definition, not because patients never feel discomfort after taking a remedy.

Homeopaths also see much more serious risks than side effects. Miranda Castro states, "In the same way that homeopathy can cure— dramatically and permanently in many cases—it can also cause harm. James Tyler Kent said that he would rather share a room with a nest of vipers than be subjected to the administrations of an inexperienced homeopath!"[34] In a few instances, homeopathic remedies are blamed for the death of the patient. (1) Some practitioners claim that homeopathic remedies can be used for euthanasia.[35] (2) In 2002, a report attributed a fatality to the patient's taking three pellets of Arsenicum 6X three times a day for about two and a half months.[36] Chemical poisonings from taking homeopathic remedies are extremely unlikely because remedies made from toxic materials are restricted by the HPUS to higher dilutions. For instance, most over-the-counter arsenic remedies must have a potency of 6X or higher, which means they are one million times more dilute than the original substance. (Prescription arsenic remedies are permitted to be as concentrated as 3X.) In the case just cited, the material dose of arsenic was too small by a factor of roughly a few thousand to be the cause of death. Therefore, the authors of the report suggested that the mechanism was homeopathic—excessive repetition of a remedy, resulting in a fatal unintentional proving.

Ordinary medicines must pass tests proving that they are effective and safe, and any side effects must be determined. Homeopaths correctly state that their remedies are FDA (Food and Drug Administration) approved. However, the FDA oversees (through the HPUS and through FDA's *Good Manufacturing Practices*) only the manufacturing and labeling of homeopathic remedies; the remedies are exempt from the safety and efficacy testing generally required for conventional medicines. The FDA itself states: "A product's compliance with the requirements of the Homeopathic Pharmacopeia [sic] of the United States ... does not establish that it has been shown by appropriate means to be safe, effective, and not misbranded for its intended use."[37]

Why aren't homeopathic remedies available only by prescription, and why don't they always carry warning labels? Homeopaths and pharmacists successfully lobbied against such restrictions in the past, primarily out of genuine concern that the healing power of homeopathy should be as widely available as possible, but probably out of financial interests as well. Maybe the adverse effects are too rare and not sufficiently serious to worry about. Or maybe homeopaths are mistaken and the remedies do not cause any adverse effects; rather, the appearance of adverse effects is due to patient downturns from natural and other nonhomeopathic causes. Skeptics would argue that homeopathic remedies are safe because the molecular doses usually range from negligible to zero.

SUPPRESSION

Homeopathic **suppression** as defined by Wenda O'Reilly is "forcible concealment, masking, or forcing under. The suppression of symptoms refers to the concealment of perceptible manifestations of a disease condition without the cure of the disease."[38] Another definition is "the act of driving a disease deeper inward, against Hering's Laws. For example, a skin eruption . . . if suppressed . . . will appear later often in a more serious form."[39] Therefore, suppression looks like a cure initially because the symptoms go away, but the disease is not cured and will return as more intense or different symptoms in the future.

Homeopaths say that conventional medicines often suppress diseases, but they also state that homeopathic remedies can suppress a patient's illness if the remedy potency is too high, if the patient takes the remedy too frequently, if the remedy is too far from the simillimum, or if the patient is too sensitive.[40]

What is the evidence for homeopathic suppression? Since suppression involves concealment of symptoms, it is indistinguishable from a cure as it is happening; it is "the illusion of cure."[41] Only in retrospect is there a chance of distinguishing suppression from cure. The concept makes no predictions and therefore is not testable. Even in retrospect, it can be difficult to distinguish suppression from cure. If the patient becomes ill in the future, one cannot know for sure whether the symptoms represent a new disease originating from outside the body or a reemergence from within of the old suppressed disease. Some homeopaths say that a cure and a suppression are distinguishable in that the patient "feels better overall" if it is a cure. This description is sufficiently vague that suppression and cure are probably still indistinguishable.

The fact that homeopathy even has the concept of suppression is paradoxical. Hahnemann was adamant that a disease can only be known through its symptoms; if there are no symptoms, there is no disease.

Is Suppression Serious? Is It Common?

Elizabeth Wright-Hubbard warns:

> Never forget that to palliate[43] a curable case is suppression. It will involve
> you in a continual change of remedies, a sort of "puss in a corner" with
> the symptoms. It will mask the true fundamental picture of the disease
> and complicate it to the point where it will be incurable. The degree to
> which this is done by the general run of homoeopathic practitioners and
> exuberant self-medicating laymen is not realized and is appalling.[43]

HEALTH-CAUSED SYMPTOMS

In patients with chronic problems, acute symptoms may or may not arise. If a patient seems to exhibit acute symptoms only after the chronic treatment seems to have had an effect, then at least some homeopaths credit their chronic remedies for these acute episodes: "Prior to the homeopathic treatment their bodies were too weak to produce an acute response to the morbific [disease-causing] agent. After treatment, however, their overall state of health has improved and their bodies are capable of an acute response."[44] This may be true, although it would be challenging to test. An additional possibility is that this is another plausible sounding but invalid explanation for why patients do not just get better after homeopathic treatment.

PARTIAL OR TEMPORARY IMPROVEMENT

If only some of the patient's symptoms improve or the improvement is only temporary, homeopathy offers a number of explanations. One is that the remedy was close to but not the actual simillimum. It was able to relieve some of the symptoms, or offer temporary relief, but not to cure the underlying disease. A closer remedy is called for. How does a homeopath know if the new remedy is closer? He or she cannot know in advance, but if the patient improves after its administration, homeopaths conclude that the new remedy was closer despite many other possible explanations.

Another homeopathic explanation is that the disease itself is changing or the patient is under some new stress. In this case, the original remedy was the simillimum for the original set of symptoms, but now the symptoms are different and a new remedy is needed.

Yet another homeopathic explanation involves the concept of **layers of disease**. Sometimes with layers, one can only expect partial improvement. Richard Moskowitz explains, "Such compromises may in fact be the best that can be done with a totality that has become muddled by a series of different symptom-complexes accruing over the years, fixed in place by long-term medication, and thus needing to be disentangled one by one over an extended period of time."[45] In this case, after each partial response, the case is retaken and a new remedy is usually prescribed. Total recovery may take months or years.

What is the evidence for disease layering? There is no direct evidence; no measurable properties of people who identify layering. The layering label can be only attached in retrospect if a practitioner finds gradual improvement using a series of different remedies. Even then, he or she cannot know in any individual case whether the gradual improvement is due to the remedies or to some other factors.

INDIVIDUALIZATION IS NOT ALL GOOD

Classical homeopathy is proud of its individualized prescriptions, but individualization has a downside for patients. Since the remedy, its potency, and the number of doses and their timing are all individual matters, it is less likely that the homeopath will get it all right the first time. Thus the patient may need to wait, continuing to suffer, while the homeopath changes the dose timing, potencies, and remedies.

MINOR AGGRAVATION SIMULTANEOUS WITH GENERAL CURE

If the patient gets better in all respects except that one new symptom has arisen, and if that one new symptom belongs to the remedy picture, its occurrence in the patient is seen as a strong confirmation that the remedy is working. Moskowitz explains: "When such a general improvement does occur, patients developing a new symptom that is typical of the remedy last taken may also be assured that it has acted well and deeply, and will most likely continue to do so for a considerable time."[46] The fact that most symptoms improved convinces the homeopath that the remedy was the simillimum, and the appearance of the new remedy-related symptom just confirms that the remedy was especially active.

Might there be another possible explanation? What are the odds that a new symptom fits into the remedy picture just by chance? Many of the most commonly used remedies have thousands of symptoms. For instance, in Clark's materia medica there are twenty-five pages devoted to the sulphur remedy, and the average number of symptoms for each of the nineteen most common constitutional remedies is over seven thousand![47] Combine these figures with the liberal and subjective way in which homeopaths sometimes interpret symptoms, and there is a reasonable probability that a new symptom will match a remedy by chance alone. It is easy to see how homeopaths might believe that a new symptom fits the remedy picture when in fact the patient has just acquired an additional symptom nonhomeopathically.

MIASMS

Hahnemann was puzzled because many of his patients failed to respond satisfactorily to his homeopathic remedies. After more than a decade of effort, he decided that the cause was miasms that blocked his remedies from working. He identified three such miasms: syphilis, sycosis (gonorrhea), and psora (scabies, itch). Miasms can be inherited or acquired through an infectious disease. When a patient has such a block, it must first be cleared before ordinary remedies can work to cure the more obvious ailment. Since Hahnemann's time, homeopaths have found many more miasms, and many believe that cancer is the result of the simultaneous presence of multiple miasms. The topic of miasms and their treatment is extremely complex; even many professional homeopaths find the concept of miasms difficult to understand.

Thus, another homeopathic explanation for a patient not responding to homeopathic treatment is that a miasm is blocking the effect of the remedy. If the miasm had been cleared, the remedy would have worked. Treating miasms requires a different approach to remedy selection.

MIASM THEORY: THE CORE OF HOMEOPATHY OR AN OUTDATED CONCEPT?

Hahnemann's miasm concept seems inconsistent with his insistence that diseases can be known only through their symptoms and that it is useless to name them and speculate about their nature: "All these perceptible signs [symptoms] represent the disease in its entire extent, that is, together they form the true and only conceivable gestalt of the disease."[48]

The miasm concept has its detractors within homeopathy. James Tyler Kent was not a proponent of miasms, and Richard Hughes, correctly or not, "considered the topic a remnant of senile dementia in an aged Hahnemann."[49] A recently published homeopathic dictionary states: "The concept of miasm has always been controversial, even more so in the context of modern scientific understanding of disease processes. It is not accepted by all homeopaths, many of whom practice without reference to it."[50]

Anthony Campbell speculates that Hahnemann developed his miasm theory to save face: "It was introduced by Hahnemann to preserve the inviolability of his system. He had been forced to acknowledge that homeopathy was not universally successful but could not admit the thought that it was not a complete answer to disease, since he had invested too much of himself in it psychologically."[51]

A handful of miasms is not enough to explain all predispositions to diseases because there are hundreds of different diseases. Genetics, environmental factors, and the patient's own disease history explain most disease predispositions much better than do Hahnemann's miasms.

Given the scientific advances in understanding the causes of disease, the primary reason for continuing to believe in and use miasm theory today seems to be tradition rather than evidence.

ADDITIONAL HOMEOPATHIC REASONS FOR LACK OF PATIENT RESPONSE

In addition to the previous general categories, the following reasons, some of which may overlap, have reportedly been given by homeopaths for lack of complete recovery.

The remedy is wrong:
- The patient is defective, being unable to communicate all of the symptoms.[52]
- The disease is defective, in the sense that there are too few symptoms to point to a single remedy.[53]
- Provings data are incomplete or wrong.

The patient is improved but is not aware of it:
- The patient is in denial of the improvement.
- The patient is impatient—progress is too slow to satisfy him or her.

The patient is not improved because patient is unable to respond:
- The patient has a limited degree of freedom of expression.
- The patient is not adequately sensitive.
- The patient is hypersensitive to emotional and physical stimuli.
- The patient's self-healing capacity cannot accommodate much of a cure;[54] healing is limited by the capacity of the vital force to heal.[55]
- The health problem is beyond the domain of the Law of Similars; the disease is not due to an inadequacy of the vital force.[56]
- The patient is difficult to treat if not incurable, and therefore the correct remedy can create only aggravations.[57]
- There is a personal or family history of serious health problems.

CONCLUSION

Homeopathy predicts that its patients will get better, worse, or stay the same, now, tomorrow, or much later, with present, new, or old symptoms. However, all these outcomes are also possible if the patient does not take a remedy. So how do we know if we are witnessing the effects of homeopathy or simply the natural course of illnesses and life?

As explained in this chapter, homeopathy provides a vast array of reasons for the patient's not just getting better, including the following:

- Worsening of symptoms or new symptoms can mean the patient is in the process of getting better (aggravations and Hering's Laws).
- Improper storage of remedy can antidote it.
- Patient actions after taking the remedy can antidote the remedy's ability to help the patient.

- Taking the wrong remedy can result in an inadvertent proving.
- The wrong potency, or not taking enough doses, or taking too many doses, or taking the doses too frequently can prevent the remedy from working.
- Taking a remedy that is close to but not the actual simillimum can result in only partial or temporary recovery.
- If the patient has layers of disease or a miasm, then no single remedy can accomplish a complete cure.

Homeopathy's belief that getting worse can be desirable is especially interesting; aggravations and changes in accordance with Hering's Laws are considered good prognoses, indicating that the remedy is helping the patient. Many other complementary or alternative (**CAM**) health systems share the conception that getting worse can be part of getting better. So do many health maintenance products, such as blue-green algae. This commonality of getting-worse-is-a-good-sign could be interpreted as support for the concept's reality. Another interpretation is that when a treatment has little or no impact on health, advocates of those treatments need plausible-sounding "reasons" to explain why the patient does not just get better quickly.

Testing many of these homeopathic explanations is difficult because there appears to be no way to make direct measurements of aggravations, suppressions, antidoting, inadvertent provings, layers, or miasms. The indirect approach of watching how the patient's symptoms evolve feels like verification and hence supports the internal reality of the concepts; one of the homeopathic explanations always fits, but so does the nonhomeopathic explanation: Patients do not always improve, especially when a treatment itself is ineffective. Conceivably the homeopathic explanations are only plausible-sounding excuses to explain why patients do not always just get better. Homeopaths clearly believe in their explanations. They are not dishonest or fraudulent excuses, but they have no externally verifiable reality.

NOTES

1. Maesimund Panos and Jane Heimlich, *Homeopathic Medicine at Home* (Los Angeles: J. P. Tarcher, 1980), p. 25.

2. George Vithoulkas, *The Science of Homeopathy* (New York: Grove Press, 1980), p. 228.

3. Edzard Ernst, editor, *The Desktop Guide to Complementary and Alternative Medicine: An Evidence-Based Approach* (Edinburgh: Mosby, 2001), p. 55; M.

E. Hyland and G. T. Lewith, "Oscillatory Effects in a Homeopathic Clinical Trial: An Explanation Using Complexity Theory, and Implications for Clinical Practice," *Homeopathy* (formerly *British Homeopathic Journal*) 91, no. 3 (2002): 145–49.

4. George Vithoulkas, I. Bachas, and S. Paterakis, "Aggravations of the Symptoms After the Indicated Homeopathic Remedy," *Hahnemannian Gleanings* 45 (1978): 175–76.

5. Vithoulkas, *Science of Homeopathy*, p. 297.

6. George Vithoulkas, "Homeopathic Treatment of Chronic Headache: A Critique," *Homeopathy* 91, no. 1 (2002): 32–34.

7. S. Grabia and Edzard Ernst, "Homeopathic Aggravations: A Systematic Review of Randomized, Placebo-Controlled Clinical Trials," *Homeopathy* 92, no. 2 (2003): 92–98.

8. Richard Moskowitz, *Resonance: The Homeopathic Point of View* (http://www.Xlibris.com, Xlibris Corporation, 2000), p. 65.

9. Vithoulkas, *Science of Homeopathy*, p. 265.

10. Ibid.

11. Stephen Cummings with Dana Ullman, *Everybody's Guide to Homeopathic Medicines* (New York: Jeremy P. Tarcher/Putnam, 1997), p. 35.

12. Timothy Dooley, *Homeopathy: Beyond Flat Earth Medicine* (San Diego: Timing Publications, 1995), p. 64.

13. David Sollars, *The Complete Idiot's Guide to Homeopathy* (Indianapolis: Alpha Books, 2002), p. 269.

14. Abdur Rehman, *Encyclopedia of Remedy Relationships in Homeopathy* (Heidelberg: Karl F. Haug Verlag, 1997), p. 160.

15. Ibid., p. 107.

16. Vithoulkas, *Science of Homeopathy*, p. 264.

17. Ullman and Reichenberg-Ullman, *The Patient's Guide to Homeopathic Medicine* (Edmonds, Wash.: Picnic Point Press, 1995), p. 60.

18. Miranda Castro, *The Complete Book of Homeopathy* (New York: St. Martin's Press, 1990), p. 28.

19. Moskowitz, p. 65.

20. Ibid.

21. Luc De Schepper, "LM Potencies: One of the Hidden Treasures of the Sixth Edition of the *Organon*," *British Homeopathic Journal* 88 (1999): 128–32.

22. Ullman and Reichenberg-Ullman, p. 61.

23. Wayne Jonas and Jennifer Jacobs, *Healing with Homeopathy: The Doctors' Guide* (New York: Warner Books, 1996), p. 129.

24. Harald Walach, "Response to Vithoulkas: Homeopathic Fantasies About Science, a Meta-Critique," *Homeopathy* 91, no. 1 (2002): 35–39.

25. Steven Kayne, *Homeopathic Pharmacy* (New York: Churchill Livingstone, 1997), p. 106.

26. Jeremy Swayne, *Homeopathic Method* (London: Churchill Livingstone, 1998), p. 107.

27. Jonas and Jacobs, pp. 18–19.

28. Cummings, p. 14.

29. Anthony Campbell, *Homeopathy in Perspective,* chapter 7 [online], http://www. accampbell.uklinux.net/homeopathy/index.html [March 11, 2002], p. 6.

30. Dana Ullman, *The Consumer's Guide to Homeopathy* (New York: G. P. Putnam's Sons, 1995), p. 19.

31. André Saine, *Seminar Homeopathy: The Method* (Eindhoven, Netherlands: Lutra Services B. V., 2000), p. 2.

32. Vithoulkas, *Science of Homeopathy*, p. 216.

33. Ullman and Reichenberg-Ullman, p. 49.

34. Castro, p. 17.

35. Elizabeth Wright-Hubbard, *A Brief Study Course in Homeopathy* (St. Louis: Formur, 1997), p. 46; Animal Natural Health Center, "Learn Veterinary Homeopathy at Home or on the Road!" [online], http://www.drpitcairn.com/Training/tapes.html [Nov. 3, 2002].

36. Julian Winston, "A Possible Warning," *Homeopathy Today* 22, no. 5 (2002): 3.

37. Food and Drug Administration, "Conditions Under Which Homeopathic Drugs May Be Marketed," *Compliance Policy Guides*, chapter 32, Guide 7132.15, (Washington, D.C.: FDA, 1988), pp. 1–7.

38. Samuel Hahnemann, glossary, *Organon of the Medical Art*, 6th ed., edited and annotated by Wenda O'Reilly (Redmond, Wash.: Birdcage Books, 1996), p. 354.

39. Jay Yasgur, *Homeopathic Dictionary* (Greenville, Penn.: Van Hoy Publishers, 1998), p. 243.

40. Moskowitz, p. 77.

41. Luc De Schepper, *Hahnemann Revisited* (Santa Fe: Full of Life Publishing, 2001), p. 251.

42. To *palliate* is to relieve symptoms without curing the underlying problem. In homeopathy, palliation of a curable case is suppression and hence bad, but palliation is laudable if the case is incurable.

43. Wright-Hubbard, p. 72.

44. Heloise Moore, "The Management of Acute Diseases During the Treatment of Deep Chronic (Miasmatic) Cases: An Overview of a Seminar by Farokh Master," *Homeopath* 83 (2001): 13.

45. Moskowitz, p. 74.

46. Ibid., p. 71.

47. *Synthesis Eight for Radar* (Assesse, Belgium: Archibel, 2002).

48. Hahnemann, Aphorism 6, *Organon*, p. 63.

49. Will Taylor, "On Miasms: An Interview with Will Taylor, MD," *Homeopathy Today* 22, no. 3 (2002): 4.

50. Jeremy Swayne, editor, *Churchill Livingstone's International Dictionary of Homeopathy* (New York: Churchill Livingstone, 2000), p. 136.

51. Campbell, p. 5.

52. André Saine, "Samuel Hahnemann and the Causes of Failure in Homeopathy," *Simillimum* 13, no. 4 (2000), p. 14.

53. Hahnemann, Aphorisms 176–79, pp. 176–77.

54. Jonas and Jacobs, p. 57.

55. Saine, p. 13.

56. Ibid.

57. Paraphrased Vithoulkas, "Debate: Homeopathy of Chronic Headache," pp. 186–88.

8. Nonremedy Healing Mechanisms

Based on their personal experiences, homeopaths estimate that between 20 and 80 percent of their patients improve after treatment.[1] The patient and the homeopath believe that the remedy caused the improvement. While it is necessary for a cause to precede its effect, clearly timing is not sufficient evidence of a cause/effect relationship; we should at least consider possible alternative explanations.

This issue will be addressed by answering two questions: (1) Is there any way to explain the improvements witnessed by homeopaths if the remedy itself is not the cause? (2) Do clinical studies support the notion that the remedy causes improved health? The first question is dealt with in this chapter and the second in chapter 11.

Homeopaths often say that the skeptics' only explanation for patients' feeling better after homeopathic care is the placebo response, but there are many other possibilities, including unassisted natural healing, regression to the mean, concurrent or previous nonhomeopathic treatments, cessation of harmful or uncomfortable treatments, healthier lifestyles, and psychological benefits. Homeopaths are instrumental in many of these mechanisms. Thus, homeopathy as a whole may produce substantial benefits even if the remedies themselves do not contribute to the improvement.

Unassisted Natural Healing

Time and our bodies' natural healing mechanisms take care of many ailments and illnesses. Since most acute ailments cure themselves by definition, most patients treated for acute ailments will get better even if the remedy is not active. Some patients with chronic ailments will experience temporary improvements and a few will recover completely and naturally with no assistance.

The Spaghetti Effect: An Unrecognized Factor

Near the time of treatment, the patient may have eaten some food, for instance, spaghetti sauce, that was a good source of a particular herb or amino acid that, unbeknownst to anyone at the time, was a cure for the patient's ailment. Thus, the patient got well after receiving the treatment, but it was the spaghetti sauce, not the treatment, that caused the improvement. Such unrecognized beneficial factors need not be related to food. They can also be environmental, exercise-related, or the consequence of a treatment received for a different ailment whose beneficial effects on the patient's illness are not yet recognized. The **spaghetti effect**,[2] as I call it, is a cure due to a specific but as yet unrecognized cause. Although this explanation of cures is rarely applicable today, it was very important over the last ten thousand years; it was the means by which many helpful treatments were discovered.

Statistical Healing: Regression to the Mean

Suppose that a basketball player averages twenty points a game. That means he sometimes scores nine points, and sometimes thirty-five, but the average is twenty. In a particular game he plays "poorly" and scores only seven points. With no extra coaching and no changes in his shooting strategy, he is likely to score more in his next game, merely due to the law of averages. Similarly, if a person averages an "eight" on a zero to ten health scale and just had several "two" days, he is likely to feel better in the next few days with no interventions.

Most patients have symptoms whose severity fluctuates. Because such patients are more likely to seek help when their symptoms are most severe, it is more likely that the patient will be better than worse after being treated (see figure 8.1). This improvement is simply due to the law of averages. If a patient feels worse than average when seeking treatment, he or she is likely to feel better than average after treatment.

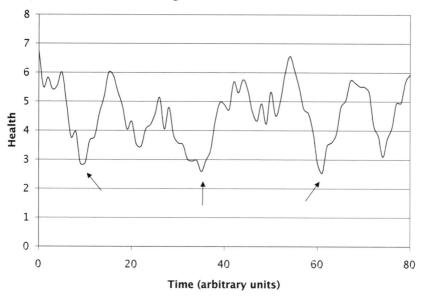

Figure 8.1. Regression to the mean. This curve was computed using a random number generator followed by some adjacent-point averaging. It is clear that a patient who seeks help when his or her health is worst (marked by arrows on the graph) will usually be better shortly afterward and the improvement can appear to result from the intervention.

NONHOMEOPATHIC TREATMENTS

Cures attributed to homeopathic remedies sometimes result from other treatments. Some patients may have tried conventional treatment and been discouraged or impatient with the recovery process. Some patients will simultaneously be seeing another alternative medicine practitioner. When recovery follows homeopathic treatment, the homeopathic remedy may be given the credit even though one of the other conventional or alternative treatments may be the cause. It is impossible for the patient or the homeopath to tell which treatment, if any, was the true cause, but it is human nature to assume, rightly or wrongly, that the most recent treatment was responsible.

Sometimes simultaneous treatments are initiated by the homeopath. Four examples follow:

1. Wayne Jonas and Jennifer Jacobs state, "If someone is having severe ear pain, for example, it doesn't hurt to take a dose of aspirin or acetaminophen to reduce the pain a bit while waiting for the remedy to work."[3] This advice makes sense, but with two interventions, it will not be clear which should get more credit for any subsequent improvement.

2. Jonas and Jacobs continue: "For most minor injuries, application of a cold compress along with oral Arnica is effective in preventing serious bruising and greatly speeding recovery."[4] However, icing alone is often effective.

3. For emotional and mental problems, Miranda Castro recommends careful determination of the correct homeopathic remedy and also specifies the following concurrent nonhomeopathic care:

> If you have "anxiety, depression, exam nerves, irritability from loss of sleep, and so on,
>
> • Seek some sort of counseling help.
> • Seek alternative medical help in alleviating your symptoms.
> • Talk about your feelings to anyone who will listen.
> • Write about what you are going through.
> • Try to understand what is happening rather than fight it.
> • Don't cut yourself off from friends and family. You need them now more than ever, even though your behavior may be pushing them away. Tell them what you are going through and ask for their help."[5]

This is excellent and conventional advice. If followed, it could well be the cause of any cure.

4. Another example from Castro involves treatment of tennis elbow: "Rest the joint as much as possible, use a support bandage, and don't use the arm until the injury has healed."[6] A physical therapist would give much the same advice and following this advice could be the cause of the improvement.

CESSATION OF UNCOMFORTABLE OR HARMFUL TREATMENTS

Homeopaths try to persuade their patients to stop using conventional medications and treatments, believing that such treatments block or mask the action of their remedies. The patients may subsequently feel better because of the lack of unpleasant side effects they were suffering from these conventional treatments; the homeopaths may say that the patient feels better because the remedy is now able to act. For instance, a woman was told by her homeopath to stop taking birth control pills when she started homeopathic treatment. She was delighted that the loss of eyebrow hair stopped and attributed this benefit to the remedy, unaware that a known side effect of some birth control pills is hair loss.[7]

LIFESTYLE-ASSISTED HEALING

Maesimond Panos describes his advice to a patient:

> On Mr. Smith's return visit, I give him a single high potency dose of Nux vomica and ask that he report any changes. I recommend that he eliminate coffee, which may interfere with the action of the remedy. . . . During this last visit, I talk with Mr. Smith about the importance of changing his lifestyle—cutting down his alcohol intake, exercising more, learning to recognize tension and deal with it. The remedy, I explain, can help bring your system into balance, but if you continue to abuse your body, you'll be in trouble again.[8]

Homeopaths always recommend that patients make healthy improvements in their lifestyles. Common suggestions in addition to those in the quotation include eliminating nicotine, getting more sleep, eating healthier food, and taking extra vitamins and minerals. Such changes in lifestyle may be responsible for healing of some ailments, and even if the chief complaint remains uncured, the patient is likely to feel better overall. In either case, homeopathy will claim success for its remedies since just feeling better generally and having more energy are counted as homeopathic success.

PLACEBO-ASSISTED HEALING

If people believe that they will get well, the belief itself often helps them get well. Not all ailments can be so helped; a severed finger clearly needs conventional medical attention. Nonetheless, for many health problems, belief helps.

The placebo response is real. A common misconception is that people who benefit from the placebo response had only an imagined or psychosomatic illness to begin with or only imagined a cure. This description may apply to some patients: Some people swear that they can feel the radio waves from other people's cell phones, and others say that they can feel the gamma radiation from a passing nuclear waste truck. Both sensations are probably psychosomatic. However, the placebo response is not always imaginary. It often results in measurable chemical and physical effects because it activates our **internal pharmacy**.[9]

There is no doubt that our minds can instruct our bodies to make chemicals and cause reactions. For instance, when we are frightened, our bodies prepare for fight or flight by producing epinephrine. Stress headaches are most likely caused at least in part by the effects of stress-caused chemical changes. Nervousness can cause shaking muscles and red skin due to the release of hormones. The expectation of food can cause salivation. The sight or memory of an extremely gory or disgusting scene can cause vomiting. People who are given decaffeinated coffee believing it is regular coffee and expecting a lift and become more alert.[10] People who drink non-alcoholic beer believing it is regular beer act a little drunk. The belief that a patient has taken a nausea-inducing drug induces a muscular response in the stomach characteristic of nausea.[11]

Although these examples illustrate a clear mind-body connection, they are not classified as placebo responses, because they are not related to healing. The placebo response is "a change in the body (or body-mind unit) that occurs as the result of the symbolic significance or meaning which one attributes to an event or object in the healing environment."[12] In other words, a patient's placebo response to treatment depends in part on his or her expectations.

A placebo response is not the same as a placebo. In clinical research, a placebo is a look-alike, feel-alike, and smell-alike but chemically and physically ineffective treatment (such as a dummy pill or injection) used on a control group to help determine whether the treatment itself has any curative chemical or physical effects.

In a placebo response, the trigger need not be a treatment such as a pill. It can include aspects of the setting (e.g., a doctor's office), the appearance and attitude of the caregiver, successful past experiences with similar treatments, and rituals surrounding taking a medication.

The placebo response is not always positive. The belief that one will become ill can cause one to become ill. Some authors call such a negative response a **nocebo response**. There are many examples of negative placebo responses. Reportedly, an office building was scheduled to be painted on a particular day. When the day arrived, a few dozen of the building's occupants complained of various symptoms generally attributed to paint fumes even though the painters were delayed and did not arrive at the building until a day later. There have been many such examples of **epidemic hysteria**.

An inert pill can induce only a placebo response, but active medications and treatments can have both a direct chemical or physical effect and a placebo response: The external and internal pharmacies can work together or against each other. A headache remedy may help chemically as a vasoconstrictor, and if the patient believes that the remedy will help, there may also be a helpful placebo response of muscle relaxation. If a patient is given a modest dose of ipecac, which causes vomiting, but the patient believes it is atropine, which counteracts nausea, the patient can feel better.[13] This response naturally depends on the dose; if a sufficiently large dose of ipecac is given, the internal pharmacy can be overwhelmed. Psychotherapy can also have both a direct and a placebo response, the latter because the patient believes that the psychotherapy will help. All types of health care interventions can have a placebo component, regardless of whether the intervention has its own physical-chemical effect.

Typically 20 to 70 percent of patients show a placebo response to a treatment, with the likelihood depending on the ailment, the strength and nature of the placebo stimulus, and, to some extent, on the history of the patient. We all seem capable of taking advantage of placebo healing, although acquiescence and anxiety seem to enhance the placebo effect somewhat.[14]

MEASURING THE PLACEBO RESPONSE

Most clinical studies are designed to determine whether a specific intervention, for example, a pill, is effective, divorced from any placebo boost. These studies need two groups: a treated group and a placebo group. The placebo group still receives a treatment, but it is inert. Neither the patients nor the health providers know who is in which group; thus, all the patients receive the same placebo boost and the study does not reveal the extent of the placebo response.

In testing for the placebo response itself, the only difference between the groups must be the members' belief that they are receiving the real treatment. If neither group receives an effective treatment but one group believes that it did and the other believes that it did not, the difference in improvement between the groups represents a placebo response.

While some herbal and other treatments used before 1800 may have had direct biochemical benefits, it is likely that the placebo response was the effective part of most treatments used throughout the world before 1800.

Although there are a few dissenting views[15] on the reality of the placebo response, some of the disagreement hinges on definitions, and the vast majority of researchers support the existence of the placebo response.

Research has found that the following factors enhance the placebo response:[16]

- The patient believes that the provider is a good listener and is really interested in his or her problems.
- The patient believes that the provider is truly sympathetic to the patient's complaints and that the provider really cares and is concerned.
- The patient perceives the provider as experienced and competent.
- The patient perceives that the provider expects the treatment to help
- The explanation of the problem and its cure makes sense to the patient.
- The patient has some control and responsibility over the treatment.
- The stronger the intervention, the stronger the belief that it will help.[16] Injections result in stronger placebo responses than pills, and painful injections are more effective than painless injections.

Homeopathy excels at all of these factors, and more so than most health practices. Patients feel that they are listened to and cared for as individual people; the homeopath wants to know about everything and is judgmental about nothing.[17] Homeopaths believe passionately in their practice, its value to society, and the almost miraculous power of the remedies themselves. They care about people's suffering and truly want to help. Patients are involved in their own treatment; they often decide when to take and when to discontinue remedies, and they work on conforming to the requested lifestyle changes. Homeopaths answer all questions and take the time to explain the process. The treatment itself has stronger symbolism than taking conventional pills; the no-touch and under-the-tongue remedy-taking ritual is notable, and some of the plussing techniques are quite involved. All of these factors enhance the placebo response, making it an asset to homeopathy, not a liability. Placebo-assisted healing is the gentlest, most natural help a patient can get.

The current popularity of homeopathy also contributes to the placebo response. Most patients have heard rave personal testimonials from family and friends and consequently have stronger belief in homeopathy themselves. Patients want homeopathy to work. It is a very appealing health care method; it is reputed to be natural, safe, and free of side effects. Homeopaths claim they are helping patients to heal themselves. The remedies are inexpensive, and many can be purchased at local stores. Patients can self-prescribe. Health care is no longer cold, impersonal, high-tech, too complicated to understand, or controlled by others. All of these benefits add to the patient's good feelings and, in so doing, increase the placebo response.

Homeopaths occasionally dispense placebos (unmedicated sugar pills) to patients who are impatiently waiting for improvement and have learned from conventional medicine to expect daily doses. Unlike physicians, however, homeopaths tend not to recognize the placebo-effect benefit. Luc De Schepper states: "Of course the patient has no clue that the first remedy is continuing to act."[18]

The best health-care practitioners should use placebo and nonplacebo approaches together to increase the effectiveness of treatments. Homeopaths appear to use the placebo effect to its fullest and deserve accolades for that.

PSYCHOLOGICAL HEALING

Visiting a homeopath is usually psychologically beneficial for three primary reasons.

1. Spending an hour with someone who really cares about the patient, who wants to know all about the patient's innermost feelings, for whom no detail is too small, and who is completely nonjudgmental will be cathartic and helpful for most patients. Vithoulkas says that taking a case

   is a living expression drawn out of the most intimate and meaningful regions of the patient's life, and so the interviewer must gently and sensitively encourage the externalized expression of this inner state. . . . It is of utmost importance that *the interviewer be interested and concerned with the welfare of the patient.* . . . There must be no implication of judgment on the part of the prescriber. Symptoms provided by the patient should be accepted with interest, but without judgment.[19] (Emphasis in original.)

2. Most homeopaths are more than just good listeners; they are genuinely empathetic and understand human nature. Whether or not they realize it,

they often provide useful psychotherapy for their patients. As Jeremy Swayne states, "Paying attention to the patient is therapeutic in itself."[20]

3. In most cases, the homeopath will convince the patient that the ailment is not serious and that it is likely to respond to treatment. As a result, the patient often feels relieved and more optimistic. Hope is a priceless commodity, and homeopaths as well as other CAM practitioners provide it.

The catharsis of the interview process, the possible psychotherapeutic effect, and the relief from serious-ailment anxiety make the patient feel better emotionally and mentally. Moreover, the resulting lessening in tension or depression in the patient can lead to a reduction in any physical symptoms both directly and through the placebo effect. André Popen comments, "I ordered Aurum muriaticum natronatum LM1 from Ainsworth Pharmacy in England and it arrived two weeks later. I called M. C. to say that her remedy was ready. When she came to pick up it up, she said: 'Actually, I started to feel better after talking to you. I mean not only emotionally, but physically also.'"[21]

On a more subtle level, the homeopath may persuade the patient that he or she is better even though the patient does not feel better. Homeopathy has a vast array of explanations of why feeling worse means getting better. If the explanation convinces the patient that he or she is better, the patient may better tolerate the pain. If the patient perceives no changes, the homeopath may again persuade the patient that he or she is better; speaking of the follow-up interview, Moskowitz says, "It is by no means unusual for patients who report no changes of any kind at the start of the interview to realize with careful questioning that something feels very different at a deeper level."[22]

All of this mental and emotional improvement can come from an office visit alone, without the prescription of any remedy. Some homeopaths recognize the healing power of the office visit. Speaking of the case taking, De Schepper states: "Half of the cure is established by being present for the patient."[23] Moskowitz comments, "The homeopathic interview is a powerful healing experience in its own right."[24]

CONCLUSION

The homeopathic remedy is far from being the only possible cause of improvement (table 8.1).

Table 8.1. How Homeopathic Patients Can Get Better Without Active Remedies	
Healing mechanism	**Amount of credit due to homeopathy**
Unassisted natural healing	None
Spaghetti effect: an unrecognized factor	None
Statistical healing: regression to the mean	None
Nonhomeopathic treatments	Some—many homeopaths recommend such treatments
Cessation of uncomfortable or harmful treatments	Considerable—most homeopaths will recommend such cessation
Lifestyle-assisted healing	Substantial
Placebo-assisted healing	Substantial
Psychological healing	Substantial

The first three of these possible causes are applicable to any form of health care. However, homeopathy deserves special credit for the remaining five possible causes. In light of all these mechanisms, there is no doubt that many homeopathically treated patients get better even if the remedy itself is not active.

Some of these nonremedy mechanisms require time, and homeopaths are generous with the time that they give their patients to respond. A cure can be apparent immediately, but it may take months or years or even a decade.[25] During this time the patient and the practitioner may just be waiting patiently for the remedy to act or they may be dealing with aggravations; antidoting; working on a healthier lifestyle; dealing with layers or miasms, and making adjustments in dose frequency, potency, and the remedy itself. The vital force works at its own pace, they say. The resulting delay increases the likelihood of the patient's healing because of one the nonremedy mechanisms discussed above.

Does it matter which healing mechanisms are most effective? The patient usually does not care, but for those wanting to improve health care, the mechanisms matter. Knowing the true causes is important so that future health care efforts can focus on the most functional elements of the intervention, providing even better results and perhaps at lower cost.

This point brings us back to the question of the role of the remedies themselves. Do they play any direct role or do they just enhance the placebo response by contributing to the ritual? A patient or practitioner can *feel* that the remedy was the cause of the cure; the frequent patient improvement after giving the remedy reinforces homeopaths' *internal* reality that the remedies work. To *know* whether the remedy was the cause requires careful testing; that is the best way to investigate *external* reality. The patient and the practitioner are usually the least objective and least trained for determining the *cause* of the cure in any kind of health care. Before we investigate this issue of testing, it is helpful to look first into the structure of good theories and to examine the pros and cons of homeopathic cases as evidence of remedy effectiveness.

NOTES

1. André Saine, "Samuel Hahnemann and the Causes of Failure in Homeopathy," *Simillimum* 13, no. 4 (2000): 14.

2. The term *spaghetti effect* is my invention.

3. Wayne Jonas and Jennifer Jacobs, *Healing with Homeopathy: The Doctors' Guide* (New York: Warner Books, 1996), p. 130.

4. Ibid., p. 135.

5. Miranda Castro, *The Complete Book of Homeopathy* (New York: St. Martin's Press, 1990), p. 214.

6. Ibid., p. 224.

7. Personal communication, Rachel Balkcom, 2002.

8. Maesimund Panos and Jane Heimlich, *Homeopathic Medicine at Home* (Los Angeles: J. P. Tarcher, Inc., 1980), pp. 25–26.

9. The phrase *internal pharmacy* is used by Howard Brody, *The Placebo Response* (New York: Cliff Street Books, 2000).

10. M. Fillmore, L. E. Mulvihill, and M. Vogel-Sprott, "The Expected Drug and Its Expected Effect Interact to Determine Placebo Responses to Alcohol and Caffeine," *Psychopharmacology* 115 (1994): 383–88.

11. Brody, p. 56.

12. Ibid., p. 9.

13. Ibid., p. 56.

14. Ibid., pp. 35–37.

15. Gunver S. Keinle and Helmut Kiene, "A Critical Reanalysis of the Concept, Magnitude, and Existence of Placebo Effects," in *Understanding the Placebo Effect in Complementary Medicine*, ed. David Peters (Edinburgh: Churchill Livingstone, 2001), p. 32; A. Hrobjartsson and P. C. Gotzsche, "Is the Placebo Powerless?" *New England Journal Medicine* 344, no. 21 (2001): 1594–1602.

16. Most of these points are adapted from Brody, p. 84.

17. At least two studies of patients of general practitioner physicians found that the best predictor of whether the patient reported feeling better a month after the initial visit was whether the patient felt that the provider had listened to, fully appreciated, understood, and accepted the patient's problems. Brody, pp. 4–5.

18. Luc De Schepper, *Hahnemann Revisited* (Santa Fe: Full of Life Publishing, 2001), p. 302.

19. George Vithoulkas, *The Science of Homeopathy* (New York: Grove Press, 1980), pp. 171–72.

20. Jeremy Swayne, *Homeopathic Method* (London: Churchill Livingstone, 1998), p. 29.

21. André Y. Popen, "A Case of Uterine Fibroids," *Simillimum* 14, no. 1 (2001): 58.

22. Richard Moskowitz, *Resonance: The Homeopathic Point of View* (http://www.Xlibris.com, Xlibris Corporation, 2000), p. 69.

23. De Schepper, p. 113.

24. Moskowitz, p. 51.

25. J. Sherr, "Full of Water: A Case of Salmon," *Homoeopathic Links* 12, no. 5 (1999): 266.

9. *The Essentials of Good Theories*

Humans have an innate desire to understand the world around them. Their natural urge to see patterns in an often confusing world is a reason behind their pursuit of subjects like astrology, conventional science, and homeopathic theory.

Our skill at comparing the scientific merits of competing theories has improved greatly over the past two centuries. Some theories are better than others in helping us understand the world because they more accurately portray the external world. This chapter looks at the key elements of good theories and evaluates homeopathy in relation to each of those elements.

FIVE ESSENTIAL FEATURES

Explanations

1. Good theories *explain* the realms they claim to cover by providing answers to the *whys* and *hows*. A good theory of buoyancy will explain not only why helium-filled balloons rise in the air[1] but also why air-filled balloons rise in water but not in air.

Homeopathy scores high in this category. It provides an explanation for everything that could happen to a treated patient. The theory accounts for whether the patient gets better or worse or does not change at all, and whether it happens today, tomorrow, or much later.

Predictions

2. Good theories make testable *predictions*. If the upward force on a helium balloon is due to more impacts from air molecules on the bottom than the top of the balloon, then the balloon should sink in a vacuum where there are no air molecules, which it does.[2] If a theory can only provide explanations after the fact, it can feel satisfying, but it is not very useful. The best or most useful theories make predictions that help us both to utilize the phenomenon and to discover more about it. If the predictions prove to be wrong, then progress has been made; the theory needs modification or needs to be replaced. If the predictions prove to be right, the theory is supported and it is more likely that other predictions based on this theory will also be correct. Well-established theories make predictions with confidence. Many new things can be "known" without having to test them.

Does homeopathy make predictions? Homeopathy predicts that, on average, its patients will ultimately get better, but that is all. Homeopathy does not predict when, how, and to what extent each patient will get better. Patient response is said to be highly individual—that is, unpredictable. Even when the patient's symptoms start to change, homeopathy cannot tell whether this change is good or bad; an aggravation and just getting worse are not clearly distinguishable as they happen. Similarly, starting to heal is indistinguishable from mere palliation as it happens. Aggravation and palliation are after-the-fact, plausible-sounding explanations for undesirable outcomes, but they cannot be predicted. Conventional medicine also is limited in the accuracy of its predicted patient progress and final outcome, but it is more predictable than homeopathy.

Many homeopaths agree that the results of homeopathic treatment are not very predictable. As Richard Moskowitz has pointed out,

> Homeopathy is a difficult and exacting art. Even in comparatively easy or uncomplicated cases, a well-trained and competent prescriber may have to try several remedies before any benefit is obtained, while in other cases, despite the most conscientious efforts, there is little or no improvement at all. Perhaps most important of all, nobody really understands how the dilute remedies act, or can reliably predict how different patients

will respond to the remedies chosen for them, or which symptoms will come, go, or change, and in what order."[3]

Consistency

3. Good theories are internally *consistent*. Parts of the theory do not contradict each other. One part of a poor theory might predict that when a coin is flipped under particular conditions, it comes up heads, while another part of the same theory predicts tails under the same conditions.

Homeopathy appears to be inconsistent. Different homeopaths often prescribe different remedies for the same patient.[4] Mental and emotional symptoms are important unless they are unavailable (as with babies, animals, and unconscious patients). Coffee antidotes remedies except where it does not, such as in Europe. A patient should stop taking the remedy when there is definite improvement, except when it is effective to keep taking the remedy. Potency matters except when one does not have a choice, in which case any available potency is given. Both dilution and succussion are necessary to raise the potency when making remedies, but succussion alone can raise potency when administering liquid remedies. Succussion is essential to achieving high-potency remedies unless the remedy is triturated or stirred or made by the fluxion or radionics methods (see chapter 13). Using a single remedy is important except in the best-selling segment of the market—over-the-counter remedy mixtures. The Law of Similars matters, except in isopathy, tautopathy, clinical homeopathy, and almost every other school except classical homeopathy. Antidoting by conventional medicines matters, except when the practitioner does not have the luxury of worrying about such things, as in emergencies[5] and whenever the conventional medicine is essential to the health of the patient. Individualizing the prescription is essential except when it is impractical (e.g., during epidemics) or impossible (e.g., homeopathic immunology). Provings can be done with either crude or potentized materials except when they cannot, as with most foods (for example, broccoli, bread, and water produce no proving symptoms unless potentized). Provings symptoms cannot be antidoted using the proving remedy and potency even when the symptom match is perfect and even though Hahnemann said a disease can be known only through its symptoms.

Although these statements may seem to be contradictions, homeopaths resolve these conflicts by two means. (1) Some homeopaths will claim one of the premises is wrong; those who advocate the premise misunderstand homeopathy. Those so accused will of course disagree. (2) The apparent contradictions can be eliminated by adding conditions and exceptions. This of course increases the theory's complexity, which is itself usually considered a weakness of theory (see the following section on simplicity).

Falsifiability

4. Good theories are *falsifiable*. There must be some measurable outcome that, if it occurred, would prove the theory false. This component makes good theories risky. If no competing theories can be proven false, there is one less way to determine which is the best. The theory that outer space is not empty but is filled with amazing *undetectable* matter cannot be proven false because the matter cannot be detected. The theory that Jane Doe has mental powers that make any integer you choose come out odd or even is not falsifiable because, although the outcome can be measured and will be found to be true, it is also true if Jane does not use her mental powers; every integer *is* either odd or even. Consequently, there is no way to test whether Jane has such mental powers.

Respected philosopher of science Karl Popper said:

"Every 'good' scientific theory is a prohibition; it forbids certain things to happen. The more it forbids, the better it is.

"A theory which is not refutable by any conceivable event is non-scientific. Irrefutability is not a virtue of a theory (as people often think) but a vice.

"Every genuine *test* of a theory is an attempt to falsify it, or to refute it. Testability is falsifiability."[6]

Are homeopathy's claims falsifiable? Is there any outcome that would prove homeopathy wrong? Apparently not. Homeopathy predicts that the patient may get better but may stay the same or get worse. Any of these options can occur physically, emotionally, or mentally, with present, old, or new symptoms. Finally, these outcomes can happen now, a little later, or much later. The homeopath cannot predict the details. Thus there is almost no risk in homeopathic theory because these options cover all the possibilities. But there is a small risk in the claim that ultimately most patients will get better, which is perhaps the only falsifiable prediction in homeopathy. Good clinical trials can show this theory to be true or false, as will be discussed in chapter 11.

Homeopathy's lack of falsifiability in its details is related largely to its complexity. In the development of homeopathy, whenever an outcome occurred that was in conflict with the theory, the theory was expanded to encompass the new data. The additions included aggravations, suppressions, miasms, and Hering's Laws. Simple theories are easier to test, hence easier to prove wrong, and therefore more likely to be falsifiable. Newton's three laws of motion are easy to state, and simple experiments can determine whether they are wrong. The theory that certain antibiotics kill certain strains of bacteria is easy to state and easy to test and therefore easy to prove wrong. The claim that a stock broker can predict whether Microsoft stock will be higher or lower at the close next Friday is also easy to test and therefore easy to prove wrong.

Falsifiability also suffers in homeopathy because many core concepts are unmeasurable. If the core concepts could be directly measured and characterized, their predicted properties and behavior *could* be falsified, but there is no way to directly observe the vital force, a miasm, or a suppressed disease. There is not even any supporting in vitro chemical or physical evidence that homeopathy's higher-potency remedies contain any active ingredient as there is in conventional medicine. Verification of all of these concepts relies exclusively on indirect evidence—the response of patients.

Simplicity

5. The first four characteristics of good theories are requirements. This fifth characteristic is not required. However, history has shown that when there are competing theories that satisfy all the above requirements, the *simplest* theory usually proves to be correct—the theory with the fewest assumptions, fewest separate concepts, and the simplest form. (This concept is often called *Occam's Razor.*) A rock falls when dropped. A simple theory is that of gravity; all objects with mass attract each other, so the earth pulls the rock down. A complex theory is that the rock is pulled down by invisible threads that shoot up from the ground as soon as the rock is dropped, except if the threads are blocked by something or are broken by passing one's hand under the object as it falls, in which case the air molecules above the object push harder on the object to make it fall down, unless the experiment is done in a vacuum where there are no air molecules, in which case the object and the earth acquire opposite electrical charges and are attracted. In this example, the simpler theory is the correct theory.

Homeopathic theory is complex, but so is conventional medical science. Homeopathy is complex in part because its "laws" are actually guidelines with many conditions and exceptions. Conventional medical theory is complex because human bodies have very complex biochemistry and biophysics. It is probable that any theory about human health will be complex. Compared with conventional medicine, homeopathy cannot be faulted for its complexity.

ADDITIONAL TOOLS FOR ARRIVING AT EXTERNAL REALITY

Carl Sagan, the famous astronomer and educator, listed some additional factors that help us determine external truth. The following quotations explain some of them. Comments on the applicability to homeopathy are added where appropriate.

Get Independent Confirmation

Wherever possible there must be independent confirmation of the "facts."[7]

Homeopathy is making progress here. Increased funding for research should encourage more and higher-quality clinical testing, including replication attempts by different and independent researchers.

Do Not Trust Authority

Encourage substantive debate on the evidence by knowledgeable proponents of all points of view. Arguments from authority carry little weight—"authorities" have made mistakes in the past. They will do so again in the future. Perhaps a better way to say it is that in science there are no authorities; at most, there are experts.[8]

Homeopathy does poorly here. Only a few homeopaths are open to serious debate on the evidence for and against homeopathy. The majority continue to have faith in authority, primarily that of Hahnemann.

Consider Multiple Hypotheses

Spin more than one hypothesis. If there's something to be explained, think of all the different ways in which it *could* be explained. Then think of tests by which you might systematically disprove each of the alternatives. What survives, the hypothesis that resists disproof in this Darwinian selection among "multiple working hypotheses," has a much better chance of being the right answer than if you had simply run with the first idea that caught your fancy."[9]

It is rare that homeopaths consider any explanation of their patients' progress other than the remedy.

EXAMPLES OF ALTERNATIVE HYPOTHESES NOT CONSIDERED

Homeopath [**H**]: "When pathology has reached an advanced stage on the physical level ... the administration of even the correct remedy in high potency can lead to severe sufferings."[10]

Skeptic [**S**]: Is the severe suffering due to the high-potency remedy or the fact that these patients are so seriously ill that severe suffering is likely regardless of whether they take a homeopathic remedy?

[**H**]: "In desperately ill cases ... where the desperate illness is the terminal stage of chronic disease, the very high potencies induce euthanasia."[11]

[**S**]: Is the remedy the immediate cause of death, or might the fact that these patients are desperately and terminally ill be the reason?

Avoid Emotional Attachment to One Hypothesis

Try not to be overly attached to a hypothesis just because it is yours. It's only a way station in the pursuit of knowledge. Ask yourself why you like the idea. Compare it fairly with the alternatives. See if you can find reasons for rejecting it. If you don't, others will.[12]

Homeopathy fails here too, though not surprisingly; homeopaths are self-selected to favor homeopathic theory. As a result, they are not the best people to oversee the research to determine whether the remedies are the cure. Die-hard skeptics should also not be the only people overseeing homeopathic research. Such testing is best done by researchers who are truly comfortable with multiple hypotheses.

Quantify

> Quantify. If whatever it is you're explaining has some measure, some numerical quantity attached to it, you'll be much better able to discriminate among competing hypotheses. What is vague and qualitative is open to many explanations.[13]

Homeopathy fails here. Any attempt to quantify the healing strength of remedies seems to lead to absurdities or contradictions (see chapter 6). Dose amount often does not matter. No measurement can quantify the amount of the active ingredient in remedies. There is no quantification of how much light, x-ray, or field intensity and duration will deactivate a remedy. Homeopaths may unconsciously sense their vulnerability on this issue and as a result instinctively avoid quantitative claims, which are risky because they can be tested and found false.

FURTHER EXAMPLES OF FALSIFIABILITY PROBLEMS

The remainder of this chapter features quotations from noted homeopaths that illustrate lack of testability or falsifiability. Homeopaths seem to be comfortable with claims that are not amenable to experimental verification. Scientists are not.

Undetectable by Definition

Homeopath [**H**]: "The correct homeopathic medicine acts immediately, though its effects may not be felt immediately. What is meant by this perplexing statement is that while the correct remedy will immediately initiate a healing response, the sick person may not manifest noticeable physiological and psychological changes until a later time."[14]

Skeptic [**S**]: One cannot test that the remedy acts immediately if there are no changes in the patients until later.

[**H**]: "Many homeopaths . . . believe that homeopathy is based upon a metaphysical principle that all metals, mineral and plant and animal substances have a metaphysical energy within them, and that this energy rebalances the metaphysical energy field of the patient."[15]

[**S**]: Metaphysical means "beyond the physical." Thus, by definition, metaphysical phenomena are not measurable. One can propose metaphysical theories of homeopathy with no fear that an experiment or test will ever contradict the theories.

[**H**]: "Local illnesses without symptoms, such as a brain tumor, rectal polyps, breast lumps, or cancer of the cervix often go undetected for a long time. . . . Sometimes the body generates other symptoms, along with the hidden illness, which you can notice. These symptoms often lead your homeopath to discover the illness and to prescribe a remedy which will cure it."[16]

[**S**]: The patient shows no known evidence of cancer. The homeopath then treats the noncancerous symptoms. Then, when the patient does not develop cancer, the homeopath can take credit for having cured or prevented the cancer no one knew the patient had. Thus the claim is untestable.

Patient Sensitivity

[**H**]: "Patients who have weak constitutions, old people, or very hypersensitive people should initially be given potencies ranging, roughly, from 12X to 200. The reason for this is that higher potencies can over stimulate weakened defense mechanisms, resulting in unnecessarily powerful aggravations."[17]

[**S**]: How do we know that some people are hypersensitive? Is it only through their getting worse when treated? If so, the statement about over-stimulation is not testable. It is simply an indirect definition of sensitivity. An alternative explanation for weak, old, and sensitive patients getting worse after treatment is that their health is frail and they are more likely to worsen whether treated or not.

Similarity of a Remedy

[**H**]: "The strength of dose and repetition needed in order to effect a change are in inverse proportion to similarity. This is why poorer prescriptions often need to be repeated frequently (and in lower potency)."[18] The simillimum is "the remedy that most closely corresponds to the totality of symptoms . . . , and when found, is always curative."[19]

[**S**]: To test either of these statements, it would be necessary to know the degree of similarity of the remedy to the patient's symptoms before it is given to the patient. However, the only way that homeopaths know with any degree of certainty the degree of similarity of a remedy is by watching how the patient responds. The logic of these statements is circular and therefore untestable.

The Deepness of a Remedy

[H]: "These high potency remedies are not dangerous in the traditional sense of toxicology. They are simply deeper-acting medicines which have the potential to create a healing crisis—that is, an increase in superficial symptoms (often skin symptoms) as the homeopathic medicine stimulates the person's deeper internal health."[20]

[S]: When a patient gets worse, his homeopath will sometimes say that the remedy has gone too deep. That may be, but what does *deep* mean? How is it measured? It apparently means that the patient gets worse on the way to getting better or has a healing crisis. One then cannot logically conclude that deepness causes a healing crisis if the occurrence of a healing crisis is the only indication of deepness.

THE LAW OF SIMILARS: HOW SOUND IS THE THEORY?

Homeopaths feel they have plenty of evidence on the law of similars, but the poor quality of provings data and the inadequate evidence that remedies are the cause of cures (chapters 10 and 11) do not meet contemporary scientific standards. Let us look for evidence outside homeopathy and consider whether the law satisfies the criteria of good scientific theories.

Before Hahnemann formulated homeopathy, he is said to have been influenced by the correspondence between the symptoms of malaria and cinchona bark administered to healthy people and between syphilis symptoms and those of mercury poisoning. The latter correspondence may exist but for a mundane reason. Syphilis has so many symptoms that "it is sometimes called "the great imitator of diseases."[21] For this reason, it may be unremarkable even if the symptoms of mercury poisoning are among the symptoms of syphilis. Some people have also expressed doubt about the claimed similarity between malaria symptoms and cinchona bark symptoms.[22] After two centuries, the number of symptoms listed for cinchona (China officinalis) and mercury (Mercurius) are 5,738 and 7,588, respectively.[23] Virtually every illness will have some symptoms in common with such large remedies. Coincidence and other factors need to be ruled out before accepting these examples as evidence for the Law of Similars.

One homeopathic justification for the effectiveness of very dilute remedies is the *Arndt-Schultz Law*,[24] which states that for every drug small doses stimulate, medium doses inhibit, and large doses are lethal. While this is true for some substances,[25] it is not a law (proven and with no exceptions) but an idea or hypothesis deserving of continuing research; exceptions are likely. The "law" does not apply to homeopathy for two reasons: (1) For dilutions past the molecular limit, the law is not applicable since it deals with molecular doses; (2) In homeopathy, the small (dilute) doses do not stimulate unless they have also been succussed, and succussion is not part of the Arndt-Schultz Law. There is current scientific interest in the closely related concept of **hormesis**,[26] the notion that small doses of substances can have the opposite effects of large doses. But the same two objections apply.

Skeptics might point to what seem like counterexamples to the Law of Similars outside of homeopathy. Many substances, at least in normal doses, do not induce the symptoms in healthy people that they can alleviate in sick people. Aspirin does not induce headaches in healthy people, decongestants taken by healthy people do not cause congestion, and penicillin does not cause body temperature to rise in well people. Also, xenon, gold, broccoli, and water are homeopathic remedies but have no pharmacological effect on healthy people (in reasonable crude doses).

The apparent conflict between these examples and homeopaths' view of the Law of Similars arises in part because the law as usually stated is unclear or incomplete and hence easily misunderstood.

It is instructive to compare five versions of the Law of Similars.

1. *Abbreviated homeopathic version: Similia similibus curentur*, or like cures like, or let like cure like.

   This version is often found in pamphlets and short books designed for the public. It suggests that like *always* cures like, which all homeopaths know is not true. This version is probably a source of misunderstanding for some of the public.

2. *Strong version* (not what homeopaths intend): Any material always cures any person who has any (or alternatively all) of the symptoms the material invariably induces in every healthy person.

   This version is unconditional; it does not say maybe or sometimes.

There are no exceptions; homeopathic remedies work every time
with everyone. This is not what homeopaths mean by the Law of
Similars, but it is the epitome of a testable (falsifiable) statement
which is full of risk because a single exception disproves it. Unfortunately no type of health practice is this simple to state or to test.

3. *Standard homeopathic version*: "A substance is capable of curing a
sick person of the same symptoms it is capable of producing in a
healthy person."[27]

This version is homeopathically accurate but too brief to communicate its true meaning. It has an essential qualification, "is capable
of." It doesn't work all the time, and it doesn't work for everyone.

4. *Reworded homeopathic version*: Sometimes some patients get well
when they take a remedy which, when given to healthy people sometimes induces some of the patient's symptoms.

This version's meaning is the same as version 3, but the rewording
conveys the weakness of the principle. The details behind the qualification "is capable of" are staggering in number and complexity,
as outlined in version 5.

5. *Homeopathic version with more details*: Some materials, if prepared
and administered in the proper way, sometimes reduce some of the same
symptoms in unwell patients that they sometimes induce in some healthy
people. Since many remedies include some of the patient's symptoms and
no remedy includes them all, identifying "the simillimum" is not possible
with any certainty. Proper administration of the remedy to both provers and
patients is affected by the potency selected, the number of doses, the frequency of dosing, and dozens of remedy-storage and remedy-taking
details, for which there are no rigid rules. Dozens of patient and prover
behaviors can (but may not) prevent remedies from working after they have
been taken. Patient response can (but may not) be additionally confounded
by miasms, suppression, aggravation, and inadvertent provings. Neither
provers nor patients will respond if they are not sensitive to the remedy. For
those who do respond, each prover gets only a few of the remedy's symptoms, and patients may find relief from only a few of their symptoms.

The Law of Similars, then, is not a statement of what will happen but only of what might happen. This more complete statement of the Law of Similars has so many conditions and qualifications as to be almost empty of testable claims; it can be seen as containing many reasons (or excuses) for failure. Clearly, the Law of Similars is not a law but only a guideline at best; laws in science make falsifiable predictions and have been verified repeatedly and unambiguously with no known exceptions. Some homeopaths are aware of this distinction and believe that the term *similia principle* should be used in place of the Law of Similars. A dictionary edited by homeopath Jeremy Swayne states: "The 'Law of Similars' is used synonymously with similia principle, but the latter is preferred because the principle cannot be regarded as an established law in the same sense as, say, the physical laws of thermodynamics."[17]

Testing the Law of Similars requires comparing provings results to clinical results. Because the Law of Similars predicts only what *might* happen, not what *will* happen, there is almost nothing to test since it is always true that certain things *might* happen. But assuming homeopaths mean that the substance of the Law of Similars is valid on average, then with enough participants the prediction of improved health based on proving symptoms this law should be detectable. However, carefully conducted provings, wherein symptoms can be causally related to taking the remedies, yield no or few symptoms, as discussed in chapter 4. The results of clinical trials (chapter 11) do not support that patients are helped by remedies. Thus the Law of Similars is weak both in the vagueness of its statement, and weak in that it is not supported by the best available data.

The Law of Similars is also weak in homeopathic practice. Many of the most common remedies have thousands of symptoms. A thorough casetaking garners dozens or hundreds of symptoms. The homeopath will typically select only five to fifteen patient symptoms as important to the case, and usually many of these symptoms are not represented at all in the chosen remedy. I estimate that the patient often has less than 1 percent of the remedy's symptoms, and often the remedy, depending primarily on its size, may have less than half of the patient's symptoms. Thus dissimilarity usually exceeds the similarity if all symptoms are given equal weight (figure 9.1).

So how does the Law of Similars stack up in terms of the properties of good theories? It does offer explanations for patient responses to homeopathic remedies but almost no specific predictions. Its internal consistency is questionable, and if achieved at all it is at the cost of immense added complexity. The Law of Similars is not falsifiable in any of its details but

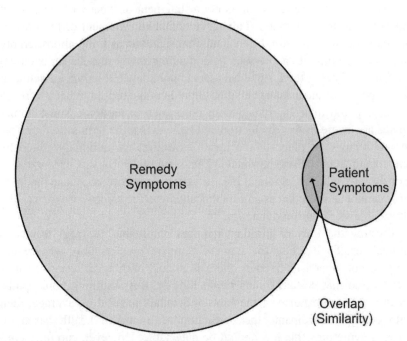

Figure 9.1. Quantitatively, the amount of overlap between the patient's and the remedy's symptoms is typically poor, which detracts from the robustness of the Law of Similars.

only in the broad claim of improved health on average. Thus the Law of Similars is a weak theory.

WAS HAHNEMANN SCIENTIFIC?

Most homeopaths have always looked up to Hahnemann as being the consummate scientist. "In fact," states one, "Hahnemann was even more scientific than even modern medicine. Hahnemann's work, the *Organon,* is timeless. Hahnemann dealt only with what he saw in the clinic and could repeat. He spent years doing research; he denied theories, most dramatically the doctrine of signatures. His work is logical, well-laid-out, and systematic. His approach is obviously scientific."[29] Hahnemann's "meticulousness" and "ceaseless efforts" have also been given as evidence of the scientific quality of his work.

In many ways, Hahnemann was an excellent scientist. He was observant and curious, and he formulated and tested theories. Hahnemann intended to base remedies on observations and data, rather than on superstition, dogma, tradition, or fantasy. Using his vast knowledge and his inquiring mind, he saw hints of a possible correlation between symptoms from poisonings and symptoms of diseases treated with those poisonous substances. Proceeding along classical scientific lines to test this theory, Hahnemann started by investigating remedies commonly used for certain illnesses. He personally ingested these substances to see if they induced symptoms similar to those of the diseases the substances were used to treat.

Hahnemann's primary weakness as a scientist was too often mistaking correlation for cause. Yes, he observed symptoms in provings, and, yes, he observed recovering patients, but he did not understand how to prove that the remedies were the cause. He was unaware of tools such as control groups, placebos, blinding, random assignment, and statistical significance. Hahnemann appropriately valued dispassionate observations but did not know that unconscious bias is unavoidable.

To his credit, Hahnemann had some skepticism about his work. He regularly used potencies up to 30C and experimented with potencies up to 300C. He accepted the possibility that 1,500C remedies could work, but reportedly commented, "There must be a limit to the matter, it cannot go on indefinitely."[30] Hahnemann also was capable of changing his mind when he was convinced that doing so was merited by his observations: A contemporary reports:

> Whilst in the earlier periods of the growth of his system he merely tells us to shake the bottle, to shake it strongly—to shake it for a minute or longer—he afterwards tells us that much shaking increases the power of the medicine to a dangerous extent, and therefore only two shakes must be used for each dilution. Latterly, however, he again loses his dread of shaking, and after once more appointing ten shakes for each dilution as the standard, he becomes more liberal and allows twenty, fifty, or more shakes, and half a dozen shakes to the bottle before each dose of the medicinal solution.[31]

However, Hahnemann changed his mind so often that one might reasonably wonder about the quality of the work behind his conclusions.

Hahnemann's stance against the dogma and tradition in the prevalent health care of his time suggests openness to new ideas. Thus it is ironic that Hahnemann himself became highly dogmatic. Hahnemann said, "He who does not walk exactly the same line with me, who diverges, if it be but the breadth of a straw, to the right or the left, is an apostate and a traitor and I will have nothing to do with him."[32]

Hahnemann also did not understand the importance of falsifiability. Faced with the failure of many chronically ill patients to respond to the simillimum, he invented his theory of chronic diseases with its miasms rather than questioning the Law of Similars. Popper describes such a reaction: "Some genuinely testable theories, when found to be false, are still upheld by their admirers—for example by introducing ad hoc some auxiliary assumption, or by reinterpreting the theory ad hoc in such a way that it escapes refutation. Such a procedure is always possible, but it rescues the theory from refutation only at the price of destroying, or at least lowering, its scientific status."[33]

But Hahnemann's most critical scientific shortcoming was not understanding how to establish cause—how to prove that the remedies themselves were responsible for all the symptoms and cures he so carefully documented.

Conclusion

Homeopathic theory does not satisfy most of the key elements thought to be important in useful scientific theories. Hahnemann, however, would not despair; he was always suspicious of theories. For him, the only important question was whether the health of the patients improved. The traditional homeopathic way to answer this question is to examine cases. The following chapter explores that approach.

Notes

1. Since pressure is higher at lower altitudes, more air molecules hit the bottom of the balloon than the top, and the resulting upward force can exceed the balloon's weight.

2. Most helium balloons will break in a vacuum, but if properly inflated they will sink before they break as the pressure is decreased.

3. Richard Moskowitz, *Resonance: The Homeopathic Point of View* (http://www.Xlibris.com, Xlibris Corporation, 2000), p. 79.

4. What little data are available tend to support this statement, but the statement is also a prediction based on the wide variety of schools and techniques in use today. See chapter 5 and appendix 5.

5. During emergencies, [Dr. Urban Mathleu] advised against worrying

about conventional medicines possibly antidoting the action of the homeopathic remedies, or about acute remedies potentially interfering with constitutional homeopathic treatment. In an acute situation, the body's vital force directs its attention to the acute pathology, and Dr. Mathleu uses every modality he has to help the vital force deal with the problem.

Kristy Lampe, "Homeopathy in the Emergency Room," *Homeopathy Today* 22, no. 1 (2002): 20.

6. Karl R. Popper, *Conjectures and Refutations* (London: Routledge and Kegan Paul, 1972).

7. Carl Sagan, *The Demon-Haunted World* (New York: Ballantine Books, 1996), pp. 210–11.

8. Ibid.

9. Ibid.

10. George Vithoulkas, *The Science of Homeopathy* (New York: Grove Press, 1980), p. 214.

11. Elizabeth Wright-Hubbard, *A Brief Study Course in Homeopathy* (St. Louis: Formur, 1997), p. 46.

12. Sagan, pp. 210–11.

13. Ibid.

14. Dana Ullman, *The Consumer's Guide to Homeopathy* (New York: G.P. Putnam's Sons, 1995), p. 152.

15. Hahnemann Laboratories, Inc., unpublished and untitled three-page document, obtained in 2000.

16. Robert Ullman and Judyth Reichenberg-Ullman, *The Patient's Guide to Homeopathic Medicine* (Edmonds, Wash.: Picnic Point Press, 1995), p. 13.

17. Vithoulkas, p. 214.

18. J. Sherr, *The Dynamics and Methodology of Homeopathic Provings* (Malvern, U.K.: Dynamis Books, 1995), p. 20.

19. Jay Yasgur, *Homeopathic Dictionary* (Greenville, Penn.: Van Hoy Publishers, 1998), p. 234.

20. Ullman, *The Consumer's Guide to Homeopathy* (New York: G.P. Putnam's Sons, 1995), pp. 157–58.

21. Richard J. Wagman, ed., *The New Complete Medical and Health Encyclopedia* (Chicago: J. F. Ferguson Publishing Co.,1982), p. 999.

22. Anthony Campbell, *Homeopathy in Perspective,* chapter 2 [online], http://www.accampbell.uklinux.net/homeopathy/index.html (March 11, 2002); Oliver Wendell Holmes, "Homeopathy and Its Kindred Delusions," an essay presented in two lectures to the Boston Society for the Diffusion of Useful Knowledge in 1842 [online], http://www.quackwatch.com/01QuackeryRelatedTopics/holmes.html [Aug. 14, 2002].

23. *Synthesis Eight for Radar* (Assesse, Belgium: Archibel, 2002).

24. H. Schulz, "Zur Lehre von der Arzneiwirkung." *Archiv fur pathologische Anatomie und Physiologie und fur klinische Medizin* 108 (1887): 423–45.

25. See, for instance, J. Townsend and T. Luckey, "Hormoligosis in Pharmacology," *Journal of the American Medical Association* 173, no. 1 (1960): 44–48.

26. Jocelyn Kaiser, "Sipping from a Poisoned Chalice." *Science* 302 (2003): 376–79.

27. Miranda Castro, *The Complete Book of Homeopathy* (New York: St. Martin's Press, 1990), p. 248.

28. Jeremy Swayne, ed., *Churchill Livingstone's International Dictionary of Homeopathy* (New York: Churchill Livingstone, 2000), p. 193.

29. Givon Zirkind, letters to the editor, *Simillimum* 15, no. 1 (2002): 13.

30. Quoted in Richard Haehl, *Samuel Hahnemann: His Life and Works*, vol. 1 (London: Homoeopathic Publishing Co., 1922), p. 322.

31. Robert E. Dudgeon, *Lectures on the Theory and Practice of Homeopathy* (London: n.p., 1853), pp. 349–50.

32. Quoted in Campbell.

33. Popper.

10. Cured Cases:
Reliable Data?

P atient response is the whole ballgame in any form of health care, but compared with conventional medicine, homeopathy gives more credence to individual cases than to large clinical trials. Homeopaths see case after case of patients who are better after homeopathic treatment. The homeopaths are all but certain that if such improvement follows the taking of a remedy, the remedy was the cause of the cure. Case reports are a major part of most homeopathy books, courses, journals, magazines, and conferences. Homeopaths tell skeptics that if the skeptics experience homeopathy they will believe in it, suggesting that a single personal experience is convincing.

Cured cases are invaluable for the patients involved; patients rarely care exactly why they got well. Cases also can suggest where research effort might be most valuable, but "cured cases" are not considered by scientists to be reliable evidence that the remedy was the cause, as will be explained in this chapter. The question is not whether most patients are better as a result of the entire homeopathic experience, but whether the cause is the remedies.

THREE TYPICAL HOMEOPATHIC CASES

Homeopaths commonly ignore explanations for patient improvement other than the remedy, as illustrated by following three cases reported by Robert Ullman and Judyth Reichenberg-Ullman:

> *Sally:* I decided to visit a homeopathic doctor after several years of battling depression. I was able to maintain an outward appearance of competency and appeared to deal with life, but inside I was fighting depression and deep feelings of inadequacy. Over the years I had been in counseling, had read all of the self help books I could find, and had reconnected with my spiritual beliefs. For the first time I truly felt that my life did make sense and that there was a reason to live. However, the sadness and lack of self-confidence remained. Every avenue of self help that I tried would help for a short period of time, but the effect did not last. I felt at that time like I was on an endless pendulum. Each time it swung, I sank deeper into depression. It was at this time that I saw an article by a homeopathic doctor and decided that I would try, one more time, to get my life on an even keel.
>
> That was the best decision I have ever made. After several years of counseling and homeopathy, I have finally reached a point in my life where I feel good about myself. The effect of homeopathy was to stop the pendulum. Finally I have a feeling of quiet peace and joy about life, myself, and the people around me.[1]

Homeopaths and patients see a case such as Sally's as evidence that the homeopathic remedy cured the patient, but the remedy was not the only influence. With several years of additional counseling, several years of caring concern from the homeopath, and several years of continuing connection with spiritual beliefs, clearly there are other possible explanations for the patient's improvement.

> *Debbie:* Debbie's health improved dramatically from Sulphur. Her vaginal irritation was improved, her hemorrhoids were gone, her premenstrual symptoms were no longer a problem, and her energy was much better. That is, until she ate some coffee-flavored cookies at a Christmas party. "A week later my constipation, hemorrhoids, and vaginal itching returned. I felt dramatically different. After feeling so good for seven months after taking Sulphur, my health took a nosedive. My energy lagged. I had headaches, mood swings, and premenstrual acne again. By mid-January, I couldn't stand feeling so bad anymore. I went back to get another remedy. Make sure those cookies don't have espresso in them. It's really not worth it."[2]

Could anything else have happened that might have caused the relapse? Holidays, with their tensions and changes in diet, sleep, and exercise, often cause physical and emotional problems. The evidence is insufficient to implicate the coffee in the cookies.

> *Doris:* While on vacation, Doris developed an acute sciatica that woke her up at three A.M. every night. The only way she could relieve her pain was to get up and walk around. Kali carbonicum relieved the pain considerably and allowed Doris to enjoy the rest of her travels.[3]

Did Doris do anything else to help, such as taking pain medications, stretching, walking, massage, or applying heat? The homeopathic remedy may or may not have been the cause of her relief.

RELIANCE ON CASES OUTSIDE HOMEOPATHY

Homeopathy is far from alone in its reliance on cases. The history of health care is littered with tonics and treatments that large numbers of people swore worked but are now believed to be worthless. Even trained practitioners, including M.D.s, were convinced. Two historical examples illustrate this point.

Revigators

Revigators (figure 10.1) were water jugs with a radium-ore lining which caused the water in the jug to have a high radon concentration of up to about 100,000 picocuries per liter. (As of 2002, there were no standards for radon in water; *proposed* safe drinking water standards have ranged from 300 to a few thousand picocuries per liter.) Because water from springs is naturally radioactive, Revigator water was promoted as being healthful because it was more "natural" than nonradioactive water (figure 10.2). Drinking many glasses of the water daily was claimed to cure most anything. In light of present scientific knowledge, it is unlikely that ingesting large amounts of radon is beneficial to one's health.

Nonetheless, at the time when these devices were popular, personal testimonials and M.D.-reported cases abounded. Here are a few personal testimonials from patients, dating from the early part of the twentieth century.

- "For over three weeks I have drunk the water from the Revigator and find it has done my eyes a great deal of good; granulations have gone, my eyes are stronger and do not water as before."

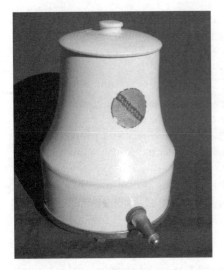

Figure 10.1. A Revigator.   **Figure 10.2.** Revigator label.

- "For a number of years I have been ailing with constipation, liver and gall duct trouble. On Jan. 21, I started to drink the water from the Revigator and the benefits have been great. I cannot praise the Revigator too much for I have been helped so much that I can eat things I have not been able to eat for years. My wife is also deriving benefits from the water from the Revigator."
- "I have been drinking your radioactive water for about three months, twice a day, and think it is the best thing I ever saw for the kidneys, stomach and for all pains or aches in limbs and joints."
- "Have been drinking water from the Revigator since January 20th and find it beneficial for rheumatism and general health."[4]

There were also many doctor-prescribed and supervised cases:

Our organization wishes to take this opportunity to congratulate you on your very valuable therapeutic radium jar. We have experienced very definite results with its use in a large number of cases. It has been of great service to us in cases of constipation and various disorders of the kidneys and urinary tract. We find that it will produce a very appreciable increase in all eliminative activities and have observed marked improvement of general metabolism under its use. Observation of our patients indicates that it is a reconstructive and tonic of real merit. One particular case of hour-glass stomach with ulcers of the stomach and duodenum, which is a very serious condition and one which is usually amenable to surgery only, has made amazing progress after drinking water from the radium jar—a really phenomenal result.

C. H. Downing, M.D., D.O.
Mina Abbot Robinson, D.O.
Robinson-Downing Clinic[5]

If the radon in the water is unlikely to have caused any health benefits, how does one explain the favorable reports? The familiar mechanisms of natural healing, placebo response, regression to the mean, and concurrent treatments could certainly have contributed. Some patients may have benefited from the additional hydration caused by drinking more water. Also, the accuracy of the reports themselves is not known.

Therapeutic Radium Mines

Even today people continue to visit mines (figure 10.3) with high radioactivity, primarily radon in the air, for therapy for all sorts of ailments. A typical treatment regime is three one-hour visits to the mine each day for one or two weeks. Again, it seems unlikely that breathing extra radon would be healthful, but there are abundant personal testimonials from patients and case reports from doctors. The following are cases reported by an M.D.

- *Case No. 5032:* Asthma: Complete relief from asthma a week after a series of Free Enterprise Radon Mine visits. H. H. K., Coaldale, Alberta, Canada
- *Case No. 5048:* Arthritis and kidney problems: "Cured of arthritis, complete relief from kidney trouble." S. C. B., Marysville, Washington.
- *Case No. 6007:* Sinusitis and thyroid gland: Sinusitis cleared. Thyroid relief: "Stopped taking thyroid tablets which I had taken for six years. Circulation much improved." Mrs. D. S., Fort Morgan, Colorado.
- *Case No. 6034:* Arthritis: fifteen years duration. "Pain and swelling eliminated. Could not comb my hair. Now painting kitchen ceiling. Two MD's had told me I would be in a wheel chair." Reporting eight months after visiting. Mrs. B. M. F., Willows, California.
- *Case No. 6122:* Arthritis, sinusitis, diabetes: Duration: arthritis, twenty-five years. "Pain, swelling eliminated. No recurrence of sinusitis or diabetes."

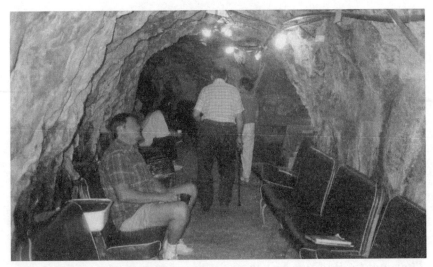

Figure 10.3. Merry Widow Health Mine (in Montana).

- *Case No. 7015:* Skin allergies: "Had skin allergies all my life. Eliminated six weeks after twenty-nine one-hour visits to Free Enterprise."[6]

That the patients felt better is wonderful, but personal testimonials and reported cases are not good evidence of cause and effect relationships. In addition to natural healing and the placebo response, other possible causes of any improved health are a higher altitude, a different diet, less stress and more exercise. The mines tend to be in mountains; many patients stay in efficiency cabins and walk to the mine. They are on vacation in the mountains for two weeks.

ANALYSIS OF TWO HOMEOPATHIC CASES

Nonetheless, almost all professional homeopaths rely on just such evidence, as the two cases that follow illustrate.

John got over his suicidal tendency, but was it the gold remedy that did it?

John: One night, nearly ten years ago, a patient called a homeopathic practitioner in a panic. She had broken up with her boyfriend, John, and he had lost his job the same day. He disappeared, leaving her a suicide note. In the note he said that his life was a failure and he was going to jump off a bridge. She was about to leave to search for him and wanted to know if there was anything that could be prescribed to help him out of his desperate state. The homeopath suggested the remedy Aurum metallicum, made from gold. This medicine is for people who feel a deep sense of failure and depression, and who often wish to commit suicide to escape from a life which they perceive to be bleak and hopeless. She notified the police and they found him on the bridge, contemplating his leap. Luckily they arrived just in time to save him. They brought him back and he was cowering in a corner. She gave him a dose of Aurum. Within a few hours he no longer felt suicidal. He continued with homeopathic treatment and became a successful architect.[7]

Some questions come to mind that suggest other possible explanations for John's improvement:

- Could suicidal people feel better after a few hours without homeopathy? Can time help heal?
- Could John's change in those first few hours have had anything to do with having caring people around him?
- Was there any counseling or therapy or interactions with friends during the weeks and months after this incident that might have contributed to his recovery, or was he just given the homeopathic remedy and sent on his way?
- Do any formerly suicidal people who do not get homeopathic treatment recover and go on to have successful careers? If so, John's success may not be attributable to the homeopathic remedy.

Here is another case that an outside observer might interpret as a failure. Homeopath Todd Hoover described treating his six-year-old daughter for warts. Over a substantial period of time, Hoover had tried a number of remedies in succession, Medorrhinum, Thuja, and Causticum, all primarily for her warts, and with no apparent effect. At some later time, his daughter got the flu and showed an emotional shift. She then was given Phosphorus.

Within several days, all of my daughter's behaviors returned to those of her prior nature, but they were highly accentuated and seemed out of balance. A dose of Medorrhinum 30C seemed to return her equilibrium. A day or two later, I noticed that the wart on her lower lip had disappeared. I found this curious, but did not make much of the change. When all of the warts began to fade a week later, I realized that we had stumbled upon the cure. Within three weeks all the warts had totally faded away. The only remnant of the episode was a small scar on one thumb where she had removed a wart manually six months before. I am unclear if the Phosphorus or the Medorrhinum stimulated this cure as they were given close together. Phosphorus is rarely used for warts, but does carry a general indication for their treatment. Regardless of the active remedy, the result was happily received. Homeopathy cured gently, completely and permanently. I do not believe I will ever tire of the opportunity to witness such a miracle.[8]

For Hoover, this incident was a homeopathic miracle, but the long duration of this saga increased the chance of spontaneous remission. The apparent failure of three remedies, one of which "fits my daughter to a tee,"[9] could be seen as evidence that homeopathic remedies do not work.

REPORTING BIAS AND OTHER SHORTCOMINGS

The accuracy of reported cases is worth questioning. Despite the best of intentions, particular facts and details may have been unconsciously omitted or distorted to match what the patient or homeopath wanted to be true. The process could be biased for the following reasons:

- The practitioner truly wants the patient to heal; this desire could cloud his or her judgment of whether and how much the patient has improved.
- The practitioner may want to succeed for personal and professional reasons.
- The practitioner may want to show off the power of a particular remedy because he or she may have been involved in developing or proving the remedy.
- The practitioner may count as a positive outcome a case in which the primary complaint has not been relieved but the patient feels better overall because of improvement in some other way.
- The patient may want to please the practitioner and therefore report symptoms in a distorted way.

It is also worth keeping in mind that we generally only hear about positive cases. Many patients fail to improve, but those cases are not as interesting to the practitioners, particularly in terms of what the practitioners like to present to their colleagues and the public. As a result, there is a bias in case reporting. We have no idea how many negative cases there were or how many remedies failed and went unreported before a remedy seemed to work. Without this information, we cannot know the real effectiveness of homeopathic treatment. In addition, practitioners may not even know about some of their failures; some patients, dissatisfied with their progress, will go to a different health-care provider. Some practitioners may count such cases as successes: Since the patient did not come back for additional treatment, the patient must have been cured. Good scientific methodology is designed to prevent problems like these.

An overriding weakness in the homeopaths' concept of cured cases is that the practitioner cannot know what would have happened if no remedy or a blank remedy (placebo) had been given. The patient might have recovered anyway, but no one can say for sure.

For all these reasons, reports of cured cases must be considered anecdotal evidence; such reports are interesting and of some value, but not convincing in themselves. This idea is difficult for homeopaths to accept; in most of homeopathy, individual cases are assumed to be proof of remedies as causes.

Conventional medicine also publishes cases but has different objectives and different standards. Marcia Angell and Jerome Kassirer explain:

> If, for example, the *Journal* [*New England Journal of Medicine*] were to receive a paper describing a patient's recovery from cancer of the pancreas after he had ingested a rhubarb diet, we would require documentation of the disease and its extent, we would ask about other, similar patients who did not recover after eating rhubarb, and we might suggest trying the diet on other patients. If the answers to these and other questions were satisfactory, we might publish a case report—not to announce a remedy, but only to suggest a hypothesis that should be tested in a proper clinical trial.[10]

CONCLUSION

For a century and a half after homeopathy's beginning, reliance on cases was consistent with scientific norms of the time. Only relatively recently has the weakness of using cases to determine cause been widely recognized; development of the double-blind approach began in 1937.[11] Not until the 1960s did the National Institutes of Health (NIH) start requiring double-blind procedures in the research it sponsored, and only since the 1980s have double-blind procedures been a prerequisite for publication in most scientific journals.[12]

Thus, for the last few decades it has been clear that reliance on cases ignores the best tools for preventing practitioners from deceiving themselves about what causes changes in health. Although most homeopaths still see cases as strong evidence for remedy effectiveness, a few homeopaths and researchers (e.g., Jennifer Jacobs, David Reilly, Wayne Jonas, Iris Bell, Harald Walach, Edzard Ernst, Eckhart Hahn, and Klaus Linde) are using the best available methodology for sorting out fact from belief. This research is the topic of the next chapter.

NOTES

1. Robert Ullman and Judyth Reichenberg-Ullman, *The Patient's Guide to Homeopathic Medicine* (Edmonds, Wash.: Picnic Point Press, 1995), pp. 76–77.

2. Ibid., p. 58.

3. Ibid., p. 42.

4. From literature shipped with Revigators in the first quarter of the twentieth century.

5. Ibid.

6. Wade V. Lewis, *Arthritis and Radioactivity* (Boston: Christopher Publishing House, 1964), pp. 72–73.

7. Ullman and Reichenberg-Ullman, pp. 28–29.

8. Todd Hoover, "Warts: To Cut, Burn, Freeze—or Cure?" *Homeopathy Today* 20, no. 8 (2000): 20–21.

9. Ibid., p. 19.

10. Marcia Angell and Jerome Kassirer, "Alternative Medicine: The Risks of Untested and Unregulated Remedies," *New England Journal of Medicine* 339, no. 12 (1998): 839–41.

11. Arthur K. Shapiro and Elaine Shapiro, *The Powerful Placebo* (Baltimore: Johns Hopkins University Press, 1997), p. 229. Although their value was not widely recognized at the time, double-blind procedures in homeopathic provings were apparently proposed and used in the 1880s. See Paul Herscu, *Provings Volume, with a Proving of Alcoholus* (Amherst, Mass.: New England School of Homeopathy Press, 2002), pp. 44–48.

12. Shapiro and Shapiro, p. 229.

11. *Clinical Effectiveness Testing:* *The Bottom Line*

From a clinical research point of view, three important and distinct questions are:

- Is homeopathic treatment as a whole more effective than no treatment?
- Is homeopathic treatment as a whole more effective than other types of treatment?
- How important is the remedy itself in homeopathic treatment?

The question of remedy effectiveness is the only one that has received significant attention from the research community and is the primary topic of this chapter. The issue is controversial, with homeopaths and skeptics coming to opposite conclusions based on the same data. The key is to consider the quality of the data. The studies with the highest methodological quality seem to be least supportive of homeopathic remedies.

EXTRAORDINARY CLAIMS REQUIRE EXTRAORDINARY PROOF

Because homeopathy's claims for its remedies are so extraordinary—many conflict with known science—the scientific community quite reasonably requires extraordinary evidence, that is, better evidence than might be required to test a conventional drug. Fortunately, science does not need to understand *how* homeopathy works in order to be able to do the job of determining *whether* it works.

POSSIBLE REASONS FOR GETTING BETTER AFTER TREATMENT

If a test is to help determine whether homeopathic remedies (or any medicines) work, it must take into account *all* the possible causes of the patient's getting better. As discussed earlier, these include the following:

- The *remedy itself* was the cause for the patient's getting better.
- *Unassisted natural healing*—the patient would have gotten well just as fast without any treatment.
- *Spaghetti effect*—a specific factor, such as an herb in a spaghetti sauce the patient ate, caused the cure, but such an effect of this herb is not yet known to us.
- *Statistical healing or regression to the mean*—since patients tend to seek help when symptoms are the most severe, they are likely to feel better in the future even if not treated.
- *Nonhomeopathic treatments*, conventional or other CAM treatments, may have been the cause, rather than the homeopathic remedy.
- *Cessation of uncomfortable or harmful treatments* made the patient feel better.
- *Lifestyle-assisted healing*—diet, exercise, more sleep, or stress reduction was the cause.
- *Placebo-assisted healing*—the belief that the treatment was effective stimulated the patient's internal pharmacy, causing the patient to get better.
- *Psychological healing*—the experience of opening up to a caring provider can be cathartic, and we usually feel less anxious and more hopeful after seeing a health care practitioner. Such changes in outlook are desirable, and homeopaths count them as part of the cure.

These possible causes of cure are not exclusive; any number of them may simultaneously contribute. Most clinical trials are designed to determine if the remedy (or other explicit intervention) actually caused changes in the patient's health.

ELEMENTS OF GOOD CLINICAL TESTING

The techniques that have been developed to ferret out cause in health intervention studies are similar to those described in chapter 4 but include some additional aspects. Understanding the reasons for the test procedures is helpful in interpreting homeopathic clinical trials. These reasons are summarized in a table at the end of this section.

Since many ailments for which we seek professional treatment will improve even if left untreated, good studies need an untreated *control group* as well as the treated group. If the treated group gets well faster or more completely than the control group, the treatment may be the cause.

Large numbers of people are needed because the researchers cannot control all the variables. Not all people in the study may have exactly the same ailment. For example, there are hundreds of different viruses that cause colds. People have different genetic make-up and hence may respond differently to the same disease or the same treatment. During the study the subjects' lifestyles will differ, with variations in diet, exercise, sleep, stress, and exposure to allergens or infectious diseases, any of which may affect the outcome. The intent is to have enough people to average out all these differences so that if on average the treated people do better, then the cause is likely to be the treatment and not one of these other factors. Many clinical trials have hundreds or even thousands of participants.

Other factors must also be considered. If the treated group is aware that they are getting the "real" remedy, they are likely to have a stronger placebo response, complicating the assessment of whether the homeopathic remedy itself is the cause of a cure. Therefore, procedures must be *masked* or *blind*, meaning that none of the volunteers must know whether he or she is getting the active treatment; the control group must be given a look-alike remedy with no active ingredient—a placebo.

Even blinding is not enough. It has been shown that if the homeopath, nurse, or pharmacist knows who is getting the real remedy, the patient may notice small, unintentional clues such as facial expressions, body language, and voice inflections. The patient may have a sense, perhaps unconscious, of the conviction of the health providers. This, in turn, affects the placebo response. Therefore the caregivers must also not know who in the study is getting the remedy and who is getting the placebo. In addition, the practitioners who assess the condition of the patient both before and after receiving the remedy or placebo must also not know who is in which group. If they did, unintentional bias might creep into their assessment of the patient's health. Studies in which neither the patients nor the professionals and staff who interact with them know who is getting the remedy are called *double blind*. It has been shown that these measures are absolutely necessary so that all the patients get the same feelings of personalized attention, caring, and hope regardless of whether they receive the real homeopathic remedy or a placebo, and so that those who assess the patients' conditions are unbiased.

Of course *someone* must know which patients received real medicines and which received placebos. At the beginning of the study, all the pills might be put in numbered envelopes. A record is kept specifying which numbers correspond to the real medication and which to the placebos. Only after all medications have been given and all outcomes assessed do the researchers go back to check which patients got real remedies and which received fake remedies.

Who gets to be in which group? If, for example, the treated group consisted mostly of believers in homeopathy and the control group mostly of skeptics, this in itself would create unequal placebo responses and consequently a biased test. Therefore, the selection of patients for the treated and the placebo control group must be random (*random assignment*).

Because random variations in health occur, so do false positives in clinical trials. By chance alone, more of the people in the treated group might improve compared with those in the control group. A partial solution is to require results to be *statistically significant* in order to be taken seriously. A statistically significant outcome is an outcome that has no more than about one chance in twenty (5 percent) of occurring by chance. *A statistically significant result from a clinical study does not mean the intervention caused the cure but only that the probability of chance being the explanation is 5 percent or less.*

Consequently false positive clinical trials are virtually guaranteed to exist.[1] Since any one study has a one in twenty chance for a statistically significant result by chance alone, in a group of twenty studies, at least one of them would be expected to be statistically significant. Studies with **multiple outcomes** are even more likely to yield statistically significant results. A multiple outcome study might monitor twenty different symptoms. That is like conducting twenty different clinical trials, and hence it is likely that one of the outcomes will be statistically significant even if the remedy is totally ineffective. It helps if researchers always report *all* the measured outcomes, including negative results.

Statistically significant results can always be found if a researcher puts in sufficient effort. Suppose that a trial tested the effect of a remedy on chronic lower back pain by asking the patients to describe the pain one day after taking the remedy, and suppose that the result was not statistically significant. Since the researchers did not know how long it might be before the remedy was effective, they decided after the test had started to also ask the patients about their pain after two days, after three days, and every day for twenty days. A statistically significant result obtained on the seventeenth day would not be considered convincing for establishing cause because the project would be seen by scientists as a fishing expedition: If one looks in enough places, positive results will be found by chance alone and hence could be false positives. With twenty days in the trial, one false positive statistically significant result is to be expected on average even if the remedy has no effect. Thus, another rule followed in the better-quality clinical trials is to state clearly in advance what the tested outcomes will be.

Another useful tool in most clinical trials is to vary the dose and look for an effect. Most people logically assume that if "it" works, then the amount of "it" should affect how well "it" works. In other words, *dose should matter*. Thus, in tests of conventional medications, the treated group is often further divided into a number of subgroups, each of which receives a different amount of the medication. This technique satisfies the need to determine the amount of medication that is most effective and to quantify any side effects. If the amount of medicine has *no* impact on effectiveness or side effects, even if the treated groups did better than the control group, then the study loses its credibility.

Many homeopaths do not consider changing the dose (in the conventional sense of how much of a remedy is taken at once) to have a significant impact on the patient. Related variables that might take its place in "dose" testing of homeopathy are the potency of the remedy, how many times the remedy is repeated, and the time interval between the repetitions. At this point, no high-quality testing has been done on any of these possible dose variables, which is not surprising. Before researchers can test these parameters, there must be strong evidence that homeopathic remedies work, in other words, reproducible tests wherein the remedy clearly causes the cure. Only then can researchers investigate dose parameters.

The ultimate test for tentative results is *replications*. For instance, if it was only by chance that a positive outcome occurred, the odds are against the false positive occurring again if the trial is repeated. Interestingly, many clinical trials of conventional medicines are not repeated. If the result seems theoretically reasonable and has some support from in vitro or animal studies, then a single well-done human study may be deemed adequate by the scientific community. If the claims seem extraordinary to the scientific community, and if there is no plausible mechanism for how the treatment should work, then multiple replications of the study will be required. If the replications are done with different patients in different geographical locations and are directed by different people, most of whom are neutral if not skeptical, and if the results of the majority of such studies are consistent and positive, then despite the extraordinary nature of the claim, the scientific community will take the claim seriously.

Double-blind placebo-controlled random-assignment clinical trials, sometimes called **RCTs** (randomized controlled trials), are considered the gold standard for determining the effectiveness of medications themselves. The key features are summarized in table 11.1.

Table 11.1. Summary of Elements of Clinical Testing of Health Treatments	
Procedure or Factor	**Reason**
Large numbers of people	To minimize the effects of any differences in the ailment, natural healing, lifestyle variations, or spaghetti effect
Treated and untreated groups	To distinguish effects of the treatment from natural healing
Random assignment of volunteers into treated and control groups	To make sure that the two groups are the same in all ways except for the treatment
Double-blind procedures and use of a placebo remedy for the control group	To distinguish the direct effects of the treatment itself from any placebo response
Statistical significance	To decrease the chance that the results are due to chance alone—to help avoid false positive results
Specifying measured outcomes in advance, and appropriate treatment of multiple outcomes.	To help avoid false positive results
Dose/response testing	To determine the optimum dose; also, if the remedy is the cause of the cure, the amount or strength of the remedy should matter
Replications conducted by different and neutral or skeptical researchers	Needed because, despite all the above procedures, bias, errors, and statistical fluctuations can occur

OVERVIEW OF CLINICAL TRIALS ON REMEDY EFFECTIVENESS

We will now look at clinical trials of homeopathic remedies, keeping in mind the above aspects of quality clinical research.

Hundreds of clinical trials have been conducted to test for the effectiveness of homeopathic remedies. Some trials are very supportive in that the health benefits are large and statistically significant. Some studies show large effects but lack statistical significance, meaning that the results have a reasonable probability of being due to chance alone. Some show a large improvement rate in the treated group but an equally large improvement in the placebo group, suggesting that unassisted natural healing or the placebo response may have been dominant. Some show the treated group doing better than the control group and yet the treated group showed no improvement; the control group just got worse. Some show no difference between the treated group and the control group. A few show a negative effect: The homeopathically treated group did worse than the control group.

The existence of positive results alone should not be persuasive because (1) as mentioned in the previous section, statistically significant results are to be expected by chance alone in one out every twenty trials or trial outcomes; thus, some false positives are likely; (2) studies can have errors or bias; this is more likely when the procedures described in the last section are not followed but can happen even when they are.

A perusal of conclusions of any large unbiased set of clinical trials on homeopathy finds both positive and negative studies. The first twenty articles listed in PubMed[2] based on a search conducted on May 3, 2002, using the words *homeopathy*, *clinical*, and *trial* yielded nine positive studies, eight negative, two mixed, and one that was not a study of homeopathy. Thus, proponents and opponents alike can find studies that support their positions. It is important to look at *all* available studies, not just those that support one point of view.

META-ANALYSES

One way to attempt to get a full picture is through meta-analysis, a research technique that draws together individual trials, both positive and negative, and analyzes them in various ways in an attempt to reach an overall conclusion.

Results

The most frequently cited meta-analysis is that by Klaus Linde and his colleagues, published in a reputable standard medical journal, the *Lancet*, in 1997.[3] Proponents seem to cite it more frequently than opponents because, overall, the authors felt that the study supported homeopathy. The summary states, "The combined odds ratio for the 89 studies entered into the main meta-analysis was 2.45 . . . in favor of homeopathy."[4] An odds ratio of 2.45 means that the homeopathically treated patients were 2.45 times more likely to improve than the control group patients, which is an impressive result. This study included four types of homeopathy: classical, clinical, combination, and isopathy.

A later study by Linde and Dieter Melchart (1998) looked specifically at homeopathic trials in which the remedy was individualized—that is, classical homeopathy was practiced.[5] It concluded that "the results of the available randomized trials suggest that individualized homeopathy has an effect over placebo. The evidence, however, is not convincing because of methodological shortcomings and inconsistencies."[6]

The problem of methodological shortcomings is illustrated in figure 11.1. A rate ratio of more than one supports homeopathic remedy efficacy; a value of one says that the remedy does nothing. The plotted points represent averages. The vertical lines are a measure of the range in the results of

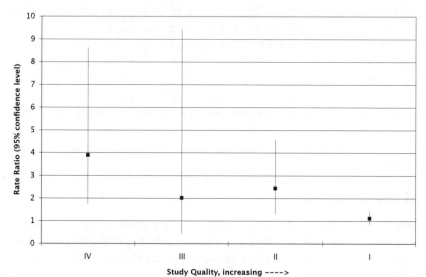

Figure 11.1. The effect of study quality for trials using individualized homeopathic remedies. The highest-quality studies are least supportive of remedy effectiveness. (Graph constructed from data in Linde and Melchart, 1998.)

the individual studies from which the averages were derived. The studies with the highest methodological quality are plotted at the far right; they are both the least supportive of effectiveness of homeopathic remedies and the most consistent in their conclusions.

The authors of yet another study (Cucherat et al., 2000),[7] which again looked at all types of homeopathy, conclude, "There is some evidence that homeopathic treatments are more effective than placebo; however, the strength of this evidence is low because of the low methodological quality of the trials. Studies of high methodological quality were more likely to be negative than the lower quality studies. Further high-quality studies are needed to confirm these results."[8]

Coucherat et al.'s analysis of quality data is shown in figure 11.2. The best quality studies (plotted at the far right of the graph) were again the least supportive of homeopathic remedies and not statistically significant. (An inverse **p-value** of less than 20 indicates that the results are not statistically significant.)[9]

An even more recent study conducted by Wayne Jonas and his colleagues in 2001 looked at just the quality of trials. The authors conclude:

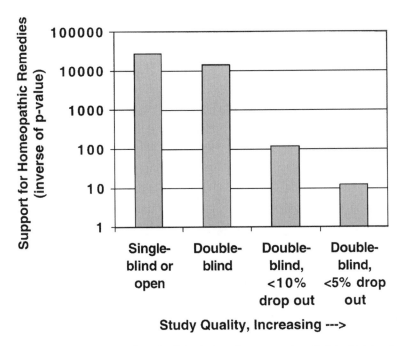

Figure 11.2. The effect of methodological quality on results of clinical trials of mixed types of homeopathy. The highest quality studies are least supportive of remedy effectiveness. (Data from Cucherat et al., 2000.)

"Compared to research on conventional therapies the overall quality of studies in homeopathy was worse and only slightly improved in more recent years. Clinical homeopathic research is clearly in its infancy with most studies using poor sampling and measurement techniques, few subjects, single sites and no replication."[10]

All three meta-analyses studying effectiveness conclude that on average, the data support the efficacy of homeopathic remedies, but the better-quality trials are less supportive, and the highest-quality trials show that the remedies had little or no effect. Apparently the more carefully one looks, the less support one finds for the remedies' effectiveness—a disturbing trend from a homeopathic point of view. The fact that the best-quality trials are least supportive of homeopathy suggests that the other trials may have errors or biases.

Although these three meta-analyses claim to provide some support for homeopathic remedies in general, they do not support any particular type of homeopathic prescribing or remedy for any particular type of problem. As Jonas et al. note, "The meta-analysis method used does not allow any conclusion on what homeopathic treatment is effective in which diagnosis or against which symptoms."[11] There are different ways of determining the appropriate remedy for a given type of patient condition; for instance, classical homeopathy advocates individualization of remedies, whereas in isopathy or clinical homeopathy, everyone with the same ailment receives the same remedy. There have not been enough test replications using the same remedy selection process and using it on the same type of ailment for researchers to conclude that any particular type of homeopathic intervention works for any particular type of patient condition.

Is there at least evidence that, on average, some of the schools of homeopathy fare better than others? The 1997 Linde meta-analysis included four types of homeopathy. When grouped by type, all yielded positive results (figure 11.3). Since there are contradictions in the theoretical bases among these types of homeopathy, and since they result in different remedies for the same patient, one might expect that they should not all work. Nonetheless, they all seem to work. As mentioned previously, an odds ratio of two means that the homeopathically treated patients were twice as likely to improve. Since the "error bars" (vertical lines) overlap, the difference among the averages is not considered very significant.

These data support three possible conclusions:

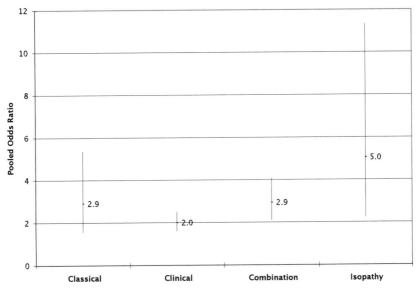

Figure 11.3. Support for different types of homeopathy from clinical trials. These results do not support the contention that classical homeopathy is most effective, but the data may be more influenced by the poor quality of many of the studies than by the type of homeopathy being used. (Data from Linde et al., 1997.)

1. If all these types of homeopathy work equally well, perhaps homeopaths should stop worrying about who is right. In Hahnemann's long and productive life, he still did not have time to explore all avenues; perhaps some approaches work that he thought did not or that he had not yet considered. Rather than one simillimum, any number of remedies may exist that will cure each case, and they can be found using classical, clinical or combination homeopathy, isopathy, and perhaps other more controversial methods.
2. Perhaps the majority of the trials are flawed; they produce mostly positive results because of errors or bias.
3. Perhaps the remedy itself is not part of the cure. This possibility would explain why all the different approaches with their different prescribed remedies seem to work equally well, and it would also explain why the measured effectiveness is smaller for better-quality trials, since these trials did a better job of excluding the factors other than the remedies.

Each of these options has serious consequences for homeopathy. Until the issue is resolved, homeopathy is in a difficult position from a scientific perspective.

Clinical Significance

In most meta-analyses, the focus is on the relative number of patients who benefit from the remedy and is quantified in part by *statistical significance*. Another relevant question concerns the **clinical significance**: How much better did the patients get? The author of a 1997 study concludes, "Effect sizes in clinical trials have often been small: In three recent, high-quality trials, for instance, the treatment effect on the main outcome measure was about 15 percent."[12] Jurgen Schulte and P. Christian Endler stated that in 1998 the average advantage of homeopathic remedies over placebos in the better-quality studies was "around or below 10 percent."[13] This percentage means that a headache that normally lasted 6.8 hours would end in 6.1 hours with homeopathy, or the intensity of a patient's pain might be reduced from a 5.7 to 5.1 on a scale of 0 to 10—perhaps worth the effort, perhaps not.

INAPPROPRIATE DATA IN META-ANALYSES

In two of the meta-analyses discussed previously (the Linde studies), two questionably appropriate clinical trials[14] were included. The results for these trials were very positive. A patient's response was considered positive if any two of the following four reactions occurred:
- The patient just got better.
- The patient got worse and then better (an aggravation followed by a cure).
- The patient had a recurrence of old symptoms (Hering's Laws).
- The patient developed new symptoms that were part of the remedy's picture (an inadvertent proving or aggravation).

It is no wonder the results were so positive. The response was considered positive if the patient got better or worse, and worse with the original symptoms or any of a very large number of new symptoms. The remedy was sulphur—a remedy with over ten thousand symptoms. This is an example of how homeopathy has defined almost any "response" of the patient to be supportive of homeopathy. These trials tested a nearly nonfalsifiable theory and hence predictably showed positive results. Only patient improvement should be counted as a successful outcome.

Proponents' Comments on Negative Trials

The following are reasons given by homeopaths for the poor showing of homeopathy in some clinical trials, followed by responses of skeptics.

Homeopath [**H**]: Most of the trials do not involve individualized remedies, as is required by classical homeopathy. Isopathy or clinical homeopathy is being assessed in many trials, not classical homeopathy.

Skeptic [**S**]: This argument assumes classical homeopathy works better than other forms, but when the results of classical homeopathy trials are compared with nonclassical approaches, classical homeopathy does not stand out as any better. In addition, classical homeopaths should perhaps stop citing the Linde et al. study as evidence for efficacy since most of its positive results do not come from classical homeopathy.

[**H**]: Most of the trials lack follow-up visits and prescription changes.

[**S**]: Trials in which follow-up visits and prescription changes were permitted have not been more positive than those in which they were absent.[15]

[**H**]: Follow-up visits are tarnished because the patient and homeopath are uncertain as to whether the patient was in the treatment or placebo group. If the homeopath thought that the patient must be in the placebo group based on the patient's lack of "reaction" to the first prescription, the homeopath might be less involved and careful in reassessing the case and therefore less likely to pick the best next remedy. A patient who thought he or she was in the control group or perceived a lack of confidence on the part of the homeopath might get less of a placebo response.

[**S**]: If this is an important explanation for failed trials, it implies that the first prescription is frequently wrong or inadequate. Even so, clinical trials should yield positive results.

[**H**]: The patients in the trials did not follow directions concerning antidoting of remedies; there may have been interference from concurrent allopathic medicines, coffee, alcohol, smoking, strong odors, or electric blankets.

[**S**]: This is a realistic burden on homeopathy; ordinary patients will have the same challenge as those in trials, so the results of the trials are realistic. One serious attempt has been made to conduct a trial in which participants refrained from all the major interfering factors. It was difficult to recruit volunteers, so the study had only thirty subjects, all of whom suffered from atopic dermatitis. The study was terminated after three years because "the evaluation yielded not even a trend in favor of homeopathy but showed impressive remissions with placebo."[16]

[H]: Patient selection biased the results negatively. Patients are randomly assigned to treatment and control groups, but they are not randomly selected to be in the trial in the first place: They volunteer. Patients with deep belief in homeopathy may not be willing to take the chance of being assigned to the placebo group and hence may be more likely not to volunteer for the trial.

[S]: (1) This statement is an admission that there is more at work than the remedy itself. (2) Such bias should have little impact on well-run clinical trials; the placebo response should not influence the treatment and control groups differently. (3) If negative expectations influence results, it is a little more difficult to explain the frequently reported cures of nonbelievers. (4) The point is just as convincing when inverted; people who are skeptical about homeopathy might not want to be part of the trial either, feeling that they would derive no benefit whether assigned to the control or treated groups. Thus the trials might get more believers than skeptics, enhancing the placebo response and giving poorly run trials a positive bias.

[H]: Tested outcomes are usually narrow in scope; they include, for instance, reduction in swelling, less frequent headaches, and reduced rash area or intensity. Homeopaths claim to improve all aspects of life, not just the patient's chief complaints. Therefore, trials should but usually do not include outcomes such as the patient having a more positive outlook on life, having more energy, not getting upset as easily, and getting along better with other people.

[S]: These broader outcomes *can* and perhaps should be included in tests although the costs of the testing would be higher. If these types of outcomes are caused by the psychological benefits of homeopathic case taking, they will not show up in trials designed to test the remedies themselves, since both groups have the same case-taking experience.

[H]: The poor results are due to the way in which homeopathy is practiced in the trials rather than to any shortcoming of homeopathy itself.[17] Only the best homeopaths should participate in clinical trials.

[S]: Then only the best homeopaths should be successful in their practices, a notion that most homeopaths would deny.

[**H**]: Some homeopaths have a general sense that double-blind studies are somehow incompatible with homeopathy, which is why these studies do not yield more positive results.

[**S**]: The validity of this objection depends on what question one wants the research to answer. If the question is whether the remedy itself is the cause of homeopathic cures, then double-blind studies are exactly what is needed. If one wants to know whether homeopathy is effective when considered as an entire package, then different types of studies are needed, as discussed later in this chapter.

COMMENTS ON CLINICAL EVIDENCE OF REMEDY EFFECTIVENESS

In assessing homeopathic clinical studies, a number of perspectives should be kept in mind.

Realistically, not all of homeopathy can be tested; it is just too vast. There are thousands of different remedies already, and in the future there could be millions. Each remedy can be prepared in dozens of potencies. In addition, there are at least millions of different treatable conditions because in homeopathy every different combination of symptoms may call for a different remedy. Moreover, there are dozens of approaches to selecting the remedy. The most we can hope for in the next few decades is good evidence for a particular way of determining the remedy for a few kinds of ailments. From this limited evidence, it will not be possible to conclude that all of homeopathy works.

Conversely, if increased amounts of quality testing with replications were to prove negative, these results would not mean that all of homeopathy is invalid. Homeopathy is so vast that it is impossible to prove that *none* of it works.

One reason for so much controversy about homeopathy's effectiveness is the small number of high-quality clinical trials. This situation is unfortunate but understandable. The profit motive fuels clinical trials of conventional drugs. Homeopathy lacks this motive; most if not all homeopathic remedies are unpatentable.

Overall, data on the effectiveness of homeopathic remedies are not encouraging. The best-quality studies show the fewest patients responding to the remedies, and for those who do respond, the average size of the benefit (the clinical significance) is small. Consequently, a number of homeopaths and researchers have started expressing doubts about the role of the remedies themselves, or at least recognizing the likely importance of other factors. Harald Walach states: "For it could be the case that the whole ritual of homeopathic case taking, treatment, consulting, and remedy prescription are [sic] powerful therapeutic agents and the homeopathic remedy would be only a kind of vehicle to convey the therapeutic effort of the doctor and to initiate the self-healing capacity of the patient."[18] Anthony Campbell adds, "It remains entirely possible that all the alleged effects of homeo- pathic medicines are due to the placebo response and other factors."[19] Jeremy Swayne states: "The homeopathic approach [as opposed to the remedy itself] is of great importance to the healing process and may often be responsible for the changes that take place."[20] Joseph Zafarty agrees: "What causes the cure is not the actual remedy given but the whole process of taking the case and *understanding* the patient."[21] Finally, Gabriella Serban believes that the particular remedy does not matter; any patient can be cured by any remedy because what matters is the particular homeopath: "If the homeopath is in resonance with this particular remedy, the patient will be cured."[22]

Some homeopaths have responded to the negative clinical trials by hypothesizing some unusual properties of homeopathic remedies and patients, for example that intentionality of the pharmacist preparing reme- dies and placebos may imbue the placebos with the same healing power as the remedies. Another suggestion is that the intentionality of the homeopath taking the case and prescribing the remedy may cause the cure even in those receiving a placebo remedy; thus no difference would be seen between the treated and control groups. There may be a carryover effect, wherein the effect of a remedy may be influenced by whether the same remedy was or was not taken the previous day. People may have an oscil- latory response to a remedy; if taken when the patient is at a low point in his or her oscillation, the remedy may have no effect. In addition, since people's oscillations are not synchronized, the "true" effect of a remedy in a large study may be diluted. Walach has suggested "a non-local interpre- tation . . . along the lines of Jung's notion of synchronicity."[23] The creativity in these ideas is evident, but a skeptic would see them as desperate efforts to maintain the notion of the activity of remedies in face of slipping sup- port from the best-quality testing.

RECONCILING CLINICAL TRIALS WITH HOMEOPATHS' CLINICAL EXPERIENCE

A dichotomy clearly exists between the experiences of homeopaths and the clinical-trial data on homeopathic remedy effectiveness. Some homeopaths claim up to 80 percent success rates and see some remarkable and quick recoveries. These claims appear difficult to reconcile with the low statistical and clinical significance of the high-quality clinical trials.

These results may not be as incompatible as they seem. (1) Almost all clinical trials have been designed to answer one very narrow question: Do homeopathic *remedies* contribute to healing? But homeopaths do not restrict their healing modes to the remedies alone. (2) Homeopaths' definition of success is eventual success, discounting all the wrong or inadequate remedies and all the aggravations and healing crises that clinical trials see as failures because the patient is not better. (3) Homeopaths may count as a successful outcome an improved outlook on life with no improvement in the primary complaint. Clinical trials have not considered such improvement a positive result. (4) The data from homeopaths is self-reported and hence not as objective as the clinical data. (5) Homeopaths overestimate their success rate by giving remedies credit for natural unassisted healing and regression to the mean, over which they have no influence; these recoveries are not counted as homeopathic cures in clinical trials.

WHAT SHOULD WE BE TESTING?

The effectiveness of the remedies may seem to be the key question, but another question is whether homeopathy as a whole heals. Do most homeopathic patients benefit more than if they had received no care at all? The answer is yes because the remedy is not the only way for homeopathy patients to get better. To reiterate, they may also benefit from the following:

- Unassisted natural healing
- The spaghetti effect (an unrecognized factor)
- Statistical healing, or regression to the mean
- Nonhomeopathic treatments
- Cessation of uncomfortable or harmful treatments
- Healthier lifestyle

• The placebo response
• Psychological healing

Since all these mechanisms are known to be valid, many patients undoubtedly feel better after homeopathic treatment. Homeopathy takes an active role in all but the first three of these mechanisms and therefore should be credited with some of the improvement.

At issue here is what one wants to learn from the testing. In the real world of homeopathic care, patients can get all the listed benefits. Testing whether homeopathy as a whole is better than no treatment is in many ways simpler than testing just the remedies. "Blinding" of the patient and homeopath is not only unnecessary but must be avoided. Half of the volunteers are treated homeopathically and half receive no treatment, and all the volunteers know which group they belong to even though they are randomly assigned. There can be as many follow-up visits as anyone wants, including changes in the remedy whenever the homeopath deems it appropriate. If a researcher wants to compare homeopathy to other treatments, he or she can include additional groups who then receive those treatments, again unblinded.

Nonetheless, there must still be some blinding; to avoid possible bias, the people who assess the patients' condition before and after the treatment must not know who is in which group. This can be tricky since the patients being examined know, but potential solutions exist.[24]

The advantage of this type of testing is that it is realistic; it mirrors the real word of homeopathy as practiced. A disadvantage is that it does not reveal *why* the patient gets better or worse, that is, which of the healing mechanisms listed previously are the most important. This disadvantage has two aspects. First, some people are curious and want to know how things work, and second, knowing how something works opens the door to helping it work better or at less cost.

If homeopathy can benefit from the indirect (nonremedy) paths to enhanced healing, so can any other health-care method. However, it seems likely that homeopathy and many other forms of CAM often have better success in this regard than does conventional medicine, especially conventional medicine of the Health Maintenance Organization (**HMO**) variety where office visits are short and less personal. It also seems likely that homeopathy does better than many other CAM approaches because (1) homeopathy's message about healthier lifestyles is stronger than most in that healthier living is not just recommended but required—patients are told that the remedy may not work otherwise; and (2) homeopathy addresses the whole person; homeopaths dig deeper into the psychological aspects of their patients than some other CAM practitioners and hence can achieve better psychological healing and stronger placebo response.

NOTES

1. Statistically significant results can be positive or negative, negative meaning that the treated group did worse than the control group.

2. PubMed, an Internet-accessible database of articles related to medicine, is a service of the National Library of Medicine and provides access to over eleven million MEDLINE citations from 4,500 biomedical journals, going back to the mid-1960s. Its Internet address is http://www.ncbi. nlm.nih.gov/entrez/query.fcgi.

3. Klaus Linde et al., "Are the Clinical Effects of Homeopathy Placebo Effects? A Meta-Analysis of Placebo-Controlled Trials," *Lancet* 350 (1997): 834–43.

4. Ibid., p. 834.

5. Klaus Linde and Dieter Melchart, "Randomized Controlled Trials of Individualized Homeopathy: A State-of-the-Art Review," *Journal of Alternative and Complementary Medicine* 4 (1998): 371–88.

6. Ibid., p. 371.

7. M. Cucherat et al., "Evidence of Clinical Efficacy of Homeopathy: A Meta-Analysis of Clinical Trials," *European Journal of Clinical Pharmacology* 56 (2000): 27–33.

8. Ibid., p. 27.

9. Lower p-values indicate higher statistical significance. Inverse p-values in figure 11.2 have been plotted to be consistent with figures 11.1 and 11.3 so that in all three cases higher values indicate more support for homeopathy.

10. Wayne B. Jonas et al., "A Systematic Review of the Quality of Homeopathic Clinical Trials," *BMC Complementary and Alternative Medicine* 1, no. 12 (2001). Available online at http://www.biomedcentral.com/1472-6882/1/12.

11. Ibid.

12. *Improving the Success of Homeopathy: Taking the Homoeopathic Knowledge Base into the Twenty-First Century, 1997* (London: Royal London Homoeopathic Hospital NHS Trust, 1997) pp. 5–10.

13. Jurgen Schulte and P. Christian Endler, eds., *Fundamental Research in Ultra High Dilution and Homoeopathy* (Boston: Kluwer Academic Press,1998), p. 5.

14. G. Schwab, *Lässt sich eine Wirkun homöopathischer Hochpotenzen nachweisen?* (Karlsruhe, Germany: Deutsche Homöopathische Union, 1990).

15. See, for instance, Harald Walach et al., "Long Term Effects of Homeopathic Treatment of Chronic Headache: One Year Follow-Up and Single Case Time Series Analysis," *British Homeopathic Journal* 90 (2001): 63–67.

16. Harald Walach and Wayne B. Jones, "Homeopathy," in *Clinical Research in Complementary Therapies*, ed. George Lewith, Wayne B. Jonas, and Harald Walach (London: Churchill Livingstone, 2002), p. 237.

17. George Vithoulkas, "Homeopathic Treatment of Chronic Headache: A Critique," *British Homeopathic Journal* 91, no. 1 (2002): 32–34.

18. Harald Walach, "Methodology Beyond Controlled Clinical Trials," in *Homeopathy: A Critical Appraisal*, ed. Edzard Ernst and Eckhart G. Hahn (Woburn, Mass.: Butterworth-Heinemann, 1998), p. 52.

19. Anthony Campbell, "Homeopathy in Perspective," chapter 1 [online], http://www.accampbell.uklinux.net/homeopathy/index.html [March 11, 2002].

20. Jeremy Swayne, *Homeopathic Method* (London: Churchill Livingstone, 1998), p. 2.

21. Joseph Zarfaty, "Homeopathy and the Search for Meaning," *Homoeopathic Links* 15, no. 2 (2002): 80.

22. Gabriella Serban, "What Is It That Cures Patients?" *Homoeopathic Links* 15, no. 2 (2002): 99.

23. Harald Walach, "Magic of Signs: a Non-local Interpretation of Homeopathy," *British Homeopathic Journal* 89 (2000): 127–40.

24. For instance, if the outcome can be measured in a lab test, the patient and assessor need never meet in person. Or, if the outcome is wholly subjective, then written records can reveal how they feel.

12. *Animals, Babies, Epidemics, and Vaccinations*

T he clinical-trial evidence on whether homeopathic remedies alone cause cures is not strong. However homeopaths cite their experiences treating animals and babies as evidence that homeopathy's success cannot be due to the placebo response. The success of homeopathy during epidemics is also mentioned as good evidence of homeopathy's efficacy. The evidence in these areas is intriguing but not persuasive; there are plausible alternative explanations for the evidence homeopaths report.

ANIMALS AND BABIES

Conventional medicines are often tested on animals before being used on humans. In the case of homeopathy, the reverse is true: homeopathy was tested and used on humans first and then applied to animals. Many cases have been reported of homeopathic success with animals and many books have been written on homeopathic veterinary practice.

One might reasonably ask whether homeopathy *should* work on animals and babies. The patient's symptoms will be poorly defined, without detailed descriptions of the discomfort and its modalities. Strange, rare, and peculiar symptoms will be largely absent. The mental and emotional symptoms homeopaths value so highly will be entirely absent. None of the symptoms will be described in the patient's own words. For these reasons, little individualization is possible. If homeopathy does work on animals and babies, either classical homeopathy is wrong about the importance of these factors or the remedy is not the cause of the cures.

Yet, many homeopaths who treat animals make liberal use of mind symptoms. For instance, Ananda Zaren prescribed Natrum sulphuricum 200C for a cat based in part on the mental symptoms of grief, suicidal thoughts, despair, desire to be silent, dullness, and desire for death.[1] People may believe animals have such symptoms, but there is no direct evidence.

Some remedies for animals do not require detailed case taking. Like some over-the-counter combination remedies for people, the intended use of these animal remedies is indicated by their names. "Anxiety" and Odor Off[2] remedies are for dogs and cats. Stop Bark[3] includes thirty-six ingredients—three potencies each of twelve remedies. Horse remedies include "Travel Anxiety" and "Pre-Performance Stress."

No provings have been conducted on animals.[4] Thus practitioners must *assume* that animals will respond the same way as humans. Why would a human remedy picture be the same for dogs, birds, iguanas, cats, and elephants? Certainly breast symptoms do not apply to birds and iguanas. In conventional medicine, cross-species transference depends mostly on the degree of genetic similarity. Homeopaths believe that people have different sensitivities to remedies; some people react strongly and others not at all, presumably in part because of genetic differences between people. But then with the much larger genetic differences between species, would not one also expect some species to have no sensitivity at all?

AN APPARENT CONTRADICTION

People are told not to eat or drink within fifteen minutes of taking a remedy, whereas animals most often have their remedies mixed with their food or water as the most practical way to get an animal to take a remedy. This apparent contradiction suggests that (1) animals are different from humans in that food does not interfere with remedies, or (2) homeopaths have mistakenly assumed for nearly two centuries that people need to avoid food and drink when taking remedies. But if the remedy itself is not part of the cure, then any way of taking the remedy would appear equally effective, and the contradiction is resolved.

Yet there are claims that homeopathy works on animals and babies. For instance, Dana Ullman reports, "Parents commonly notice that teething and colicky babies stop crying within seconds after a homeopathic medicine is given."[5] There appear to be no published clinical trials involving babies; thus the claim for efficacy is based on anecdotal evidence alone. There are some clinical trials involving animals. Overall, the results are similar to those on humans in that both positive and negative results can be found. However, both the number and the quality of the animal studies are lower; some even have no control group, so one cannot know if the treated group benefited.[6] Taken as a whole, these trials do not make a convincing case.

Certainly, some animals have gotten better after being given a homeopathic remedy, but the remedy need not have been the cause. In an example noted by Steven Ransom,[7] a cow suffering from milk fever showed improvement in less than an hour after being given a few drops of a homeopathic remedy. Milk fever is caused by calcium deficiency in the blood. Shortly before being treated homeopathically, the cow had received the intravenous calcium injection that is the standard treatment for milk fever. The cow recovered, but the homeopathic remedy was obviously not necessarily the cause of the recovery.

Animals and babies can certainly benefit from most of the nonremedy ways that adult humans may get better, such as unassisted natural healing, concurrent or previous nonhomeopathic treatments and regression to the mean. Even the placebo response is not entirely out of the question. Animals and babies certainly are capable of biochemical responses due to conditioning. An example is the salivation of dogs upon hearing a sound that, in the past, had been followed by food (Pavlov's experiments). Tender loving care and attention might help or at least be a distraction, as would the sweet taste of the remedies. The only way to rule out all these nonremedy causes is through high-quality RCTs repeated by independent researchers.

HISTORICAL EPIDEMICS

Homeopathy has long claimed impressive evidence for using its remedies during epidemics of diseases such as scarlet fever, cholera, and influenza. When dealing with epidemics, homeopaths select a single or a few remedies based on the pooled symptoms of many patients.[8] (Within a given epidemic, homeopaths believe that different remedies may be needed in different geographical regions and at different times, perhaps because the epidemic, as seen through the patients' symptoms, evolves with time and may vary with location.)

This sweeping approach to treating epidemics looks like conventional medicine, not homeopathy. A single disease is assumed to be affecting many patients, and the remedy is the same for everyone. The disease is being treated, not the individuals. Homeopathy does not in this instance look for or use the strange, rare, and peculiar symptoms that are said to be important in classical homeopathy for finding the simillimum.

Another approach to remedy selection for epidemics is the use of the disease nosode—the remedy made from the infected tissues or body fluids from patients with the disease. This approach is even further removed from classical homeopathy. The remedies do not need to be proven, and no patient symptoms are needed. It is simply assumed that a homeopathically prepared remedy made from a disease can cure the same disease.

There is reason to be impressed if the historical reports of home-opathy's success during epidemics are valid and if the remedies were the cause, but there are good reasons to question both. Miranda Castro describes homeopathy's success with epidemics:

> In 1831 cholera swept through Central Europe. Hahnemann published papers on the homeopathic treatment of the disease, advocating the administration of the remedy Camphor in the early stages and Cuprum metallicurn, Veratrum album, Bryonia alba and Rhus toxicodendron in the later stages. He also stressed that clothing and bedding should be heated to destroy "all known infectious matters" and advised cleanliness, ventilation and disinfection of the rooms, and quarantine. In such respects his ideas were far ahead of his time: the work of Pasteur on the germ theory of disease and that of Lister on disinfection were still to come.[9]

If homeopathic hospitals took these precautions to limit infection and other hospitals did not, we might have a plausible alternative explanation as to why the homeopathic patients did better. In addition, homeopathic patients almost certainly benefited from the absence of sometimes fatal treatments administered by nonhomeopathic practitioners—practices such as bloodletting, purging, dehydration, and large doses of mercury. Thus a higher success rate of homeopathically treated patients does not guarantee that the remedies were the cause of the success.

Are the reports themselves reliable? Most of the data were gathered between fifty and two hundred years ago when methodological standards were significantly poorer than they are today. As homeopath Todd Hoover notes:

The data from epidemics is mixed information. Prophylactic use of remedies is often commingled with treatment of already ill patients. Some of the data from individual prescribers appears [*sic*] to be of questionable veracity; often, the allopathic results have been misrepresented as much less effective than reputable sources have recorded. This type of information often appears more as slanderous attacks on allopathic medicine than as true and accurate reporting.[10]

There is also the likelihood of selective data reporting. Hahnemann claimed great success treating a scarlet fever epidemic with Belladonna. When other physicians reported negative results with Belladonna, Hahnemann claimed that they failed because it was not scarlet fever or it was a different strain of scarlet fever; he said that the remedy must match the symptoms of each outbreak.[11] Perhaps this assertion is true, but it may point to reporting bias: The negative results are not reported as homeopathic failures because according to the homeopath, the remedy was not properly selected. It is also possible that the claim of spatial and temporal differences in the disease during an epidemic, although not entirely implausible, might be only a rationalization for why homeopathy did not always seem to work.

Without time travel, the issue of data validity and interpretation cannot be resolved. While it is plausible that *homeopathy* saved lives due to hygiene, quarantine, and avoidance of harmful treatments, the evidence that *homeopathic remedies* saved lives is not convincing. To make a strong case for the application of homeopathic remedies in the case of epidemics, we need data from contemporary epidemics gathered with contemporary methodological standards.

Related to epidemic disease treatment is the use of the popular Oscillococcinum remedy today for flu. Luc De Schepper states, "I and others have seen it work provided it is given *early* enough."[12] If it is in fact ineffective, the emphasis on giving the remedy early makes sense; the earlier the remedy is given, the less certain one can be that the patient has the flu. The remedy is more likely to appear to work because some of the patients did not have the flu.

SHOULD HOMEOPATHIC REMEDIES WORK BECAUSE THEY ARE LIKE VACCINATIONS?

The Law of Similars seems analogous to vaccinations: Very small amounts of medication can have dramatic effects, and the same agent that causes the disease seems to prevent the disease. Thus, the effectiveness of vaccinations is often cited as evidence for the effectiveness of very dilute homeopathic remedies. This argument is specious because (1) classical homeopathy is not based on "same cures same" but "like cures like." The curative remedy produces similar symptoms but is not made from the cause of the disease, as are vaccinations; (2) vaccinations contain actual molecules related to original starting material whereas higher potency homeopathic remedies do not; (3) vaccination stock does not become more potent with more dilution and shaking, as is claimed for homeopathic remedies; (4) the emphasis with vaccinations is on preventing illnesses, whereas homeopathy focuses on curing the sick; (5) homeopathic remedies are individualized, while vaccines are not; (6) vaccinations claim to be effective for only a small percentage of all human diseases, whereas homeopathic remedies claim to be effective for almost any human condition; (7) vaccinations have been proven to stimulate the immune system, while homeopathic remedies have not;[13] (8) vaccinations have essentially eradicated some infectious diseases, whereas homeopaths claim only to treat or prevent illness in individuals. Even if none of the listed items was problematic, vaccinations would support only isopathy, not classical homeopathy, because there is no symptom matching.

HOMEOPATHIC VACCINATION

Homeopathic immunology or prophylaxis is used by those homeopaths who believe that remedies can be used to prevent particular illnesses as in (1) protecting exposed people from contracting disease during epidemics, such as smallpox and scarlet fever, (2) immunizations against serious childhood diseases, and (3) prevention of more mundane problems such as influenza and reactions to poison ivy. Remedies used in homeopathic prophylaxis can be made from the causative agent (e.g., poison ivy remedy to prevent poison ivy rash, or tuberculosis remedy to prevent tuberculosis), or a remedy whose symptom picture is a good match to the generalized symptoms of the disease. Homeopaths have claimed success in preventing smallpox, diphtheria, polio, meningitis, whooping cough,[14] and plague.[15]

Homeopathic disease prevention seems distant from classical homeopathy. The patient has no symptoms, so there can be no individualization of the symptoms. Since the patient is not ill, classical homeopathy might see such treatment as risking an inadvertent proving. Noted homeopathic educator Dana Ullman has pointed out the contradiction between homeopathic prophylaxis and classical homeopathy and does not see evidence for effectiveness of the former.[16]

Homeopaths are enamored of homeopathic vaccination because of concerns about the safety of conventional vaccination. While there is a small but real risk associated with some of the childhood vaccinations, the risk to the child (and to society) of not being vaccinated is much higher.[17] This risk is like the "tragedy of the commons"[18] discussed by Garrett Hardin. If members of a village share common grazing land, any individual stands to gain by increasing the size of his herd, but if everyone triples his herd, all the animals may die of starvation. If only one person is selfish, that person gains; if everyone acts selfishly, everyone loses. Thus, if it is only John and Mary Doe's children that are not vaccinated, their children will probably not get the disease; the fact that all other children are vaccinated decreases the odds of the Does' children being exposed. However, if many other families also opt to forego vaccination, the chance of the disease's spreading increases. Then the risk to all the unvaccinated children is high, in fact higher than the small risk of the vaccination itself. Many more children will suffer and even die; the Does' children may be among them or may be the cause of others' deaths. Thus it is selfish to depend on most other children being vaccinated rather than having one's own children vaccinated.

NOTES

1. Ananda Zaren, "Cats Don't Talk," *Homeopathy Today* (2001): 18–19.

2. Washington Homeopathic Products, Inc.

3. Natural Veterinary Pharmaceuticals.

4. Steven Kayne, *Homeopathic Pharmacy* (New York: Churchill Livingstone, 1997), pp. 150–51.

5. Dana Ullman, *The Consumer's Guide to Homeopathy* (New York: G. P. Putnam's Sons, 1995), p. 66.

6. See, for example, M. Elliott, "Cushing's Disease: A New Approach to Therapy in Equine and Canine Patients," *British Homeopathic Journal* 90, no. 1 (2001): 33–36.

7. Steven Ransom, *Homeopathy: What Are We Swallowing?* (Uckfield, U.K.: Credence Publications, 1999), pp. 96–99.

8. Todd Hoover, "Homeopathic Prophylaxis: Fact or Fiction?" *Journal of the American Institute of Homeopathy* 94, no. 3 (2001): 168–75.

9. Miranda Castro, *The Complete Book of Homeopathy* (New York: St. Martin's Press, 1990), p. 6.

10. Hoover, p. 173.

11. Samuel Hahnemann, *Materia Medica Pura*, vol. 1 (1811; reprint, New Delhi: B. Jain Publishers, 1999), p. 200.

12. Luc De Schepper, *Hahnemann Revisited* (Santa Fe: Full of Life Publishing, 2001), p. 201.

13. There is research interest on this topic but no convincing data yet.

14. Michael Traub, "Homeopathic Prophylaxis: Synopsis of Published Research," *Homeopathy Today* 21, no. 11 (2001): 16–17.

15. William Boericke, *Homoeopathic Materia Medica* [online], http://www.homeoint.org/books/boericmm/i/ign.htm [Nov. 15, 2002].

16. Ullman, p. 328.

17. "Vaccines: An Issue of Trust," *Consumer Reports* 66, no. 8 (2001): 17–21.

18. Garrett Hardin, "The Tragedy of the Commons," *Science* 162 (1968): 1243–48.

13. *The Homeopathic Fringe or the Leading Edge?*

All fields have fringes—practices and theories so far from their mainstream that many people lift their eyebrows in amazement or concern when they hear about them. Most homeopaths seem to be supportive of their fringe, believing that the diversity of approaches is part of the power of homeopathy. However, some homeopaths, such as George Vithoulkas, Julian Winston, and André Saine, are critical of homeopathy's fringes. Most ideas on the fringes of any field prove ultimately to be wrong. However, a small fraction of fringe ideas prove to be correct; thus the fringes deserve some attention.

This chapter presents practices and ideas in homeopathy that are somewhat distant from the homeopathic mainstream. I recognize that the divisions between generally accepted and fringe practices is itself fuzzy and apologize to those readers who are offended by my demarcation.

GRAFTING

Apparently, one need never buy any given homeopathic remedy more than once, thanks to the process of **grafting**, as explained by Bill Gray:

> A few granules of potentized sugar, when added to a vial of unmedicated sugar, renders [*sic*] all the granules in the vial as potent in turn—a process

known to homeopaths as "grafting." As a general rule, homeopaths do not rely on "grafting" because pharmacies need to sell product in order to maintain high standards of quality. Nevertheless, the phenomenon exists and needs to be taken into account.[1]

Both grafting and plussing purportedly yield any amount of just-as-potent remedy just by adding one pellet of remedy to unmedicated pellets, or normal sugar, or plain water. Thus one pellet of a remedy could be "expanded" to serve all humankind forever. Virtually no other health practice can get so much from so little, but then no other health practice has nonmolecular medicines.

WITCHCRAFT

Some homeopaths do not even try to approach their field scientifically. Homeopath Jörg Wichmann believes that homeopathy is in the "hermetic" tradition, "which puts homeopathy in the same line as shamanism and alchemy. . . . So let's just say: 'Yes, homeopathy is as much witchcraft as you have ever suspected it to be.'"[2]

UNORTHODOX REMEDY-TAKING

Remedies can be taken in many ways. Robert Ullman and Judyth Reichenberg-Ullman state:

> As long as the correct remedy is given, nearly any mode of administration will produce a positive effect. One homeopathic patient went to her homeopath for help with anxiety and insomnia. The homeopath prescribed Arsenicum album to be taken orally. The patient misunderstood the instructions and dumped the contents of the envelope in her bath water. The remedy still worked.[3]

In another case, a young girl had green and strong-smelling discharges from her ears. Her father picked up her prescription, Pulsatilla 200C, to be taken orally.

> Two days later her dad called, incredulous that the remedy had worked. There was no more discharge and no more pain. He then asked, "Should I keep put-

ting the drops *in her ears?*" So much for rituals! When the simillimum res-
onates, the form in which it is dispensed is inconsequential. I have had
mothers tell me that the child would not take the remedy. The mother would
then physically restrain the child and pop the remedy dry into the child's
mouth, only to have the child spit it back out. Even still, the remedy cleared
the pathology. This is a great tribute to the power of homeopathy. If the simillimum is introduced into the organism, it will have a curative effect.[4]

Even though these cases were accidents, the view is widespread that oral
remedies need not be taken orally to be effective. For very sensitive patients,
the "friction method" is sometimes used, wherein a liquid form of the remedy
is rubbed on the healthy skin of the patient's entire body.[5] It is claimed that
for treating infants, pellets may be dissolved in water and the resulting solution can be used to moisten the infant's lips,[6] wrists, or temples.[7]

According to some homeopaths, a sniff of a remedy intended to be
taken orally can be effective, and sometimes an even more abstract connection to the remedy will work. A patient who is thought to be extremely sensitive is first treated by being in a room where the remedy bottle is briefly
opened and then closed. A slightly less sensitive patient might be allowed
a brief sniff through just one nostril and then later a sniff through both nos-
trils.[8] For the most sensitive patients, the bottle is never opened at all.
Moskowitz says, "Some patients who overreact to the customary tiny
amounts seem to do better with less, or even by carrying the remedy in a
vial on their person and not ingesting it at all."[9]

Some homeopaths create their own remedies without using any original medicinal material. Practitioners draw a ten-sided figure on a piece of
paper and write the name of the desired remedy outside the figure; a glass
of water placed in the center of this figure for a few minutes will become
the remedy. Some practitioners use a triangle or circle instead of the ten-
sided figure and find that works just as well.[10] Another technique involves
making **radionics**. A bottle with virgin pellets or liquid is placed in the
middle of a piece of paper or cardboard carefully aligned north, on which
is drawn a geometric figure. The shape and size of the figure determine the
remedy and its potency, respectively. The contents of the bottle then
become the remedy. The geometric figures for each remedy are determined
by dowsing with a pendulum all around a "real" bottle of the remedy and
noting at what points the pendulum responds; connecting these points creates the geometric figure. In some cases, magnetism is used as well as
cards. Some homeopaths find that these remedies work but do not "hold as
well"[11] as remedies prepared in the usual fashion.

Reportedly animals can also be affected by remedies without ingesting them. According to Dana Ullman:

> In one very intriguing study, Thyroxine 30X (thyroid hormone) was placed in the water of tadpoles. When compared to tadpoles who were given a placebo, the study showed, morphogenesis of the tadpoles into frogs was slowed for those who were exposed to the homeopathic doses. Because thyroid hormone in crude [real chemical] doses is known to speed up morphogenesis, it makes sense from a homeopathic perspective that homeopathic doses would slow it down.
>
> What makes this study more interesting is that additional investigations resulted in the same effect when a glass bottle of the homeopathic doses of thyroid hormone was simply suspended in the water with the lip of the bottle above the water line. This research was replicated at several laboratories, and results were consistent.
>
> The implications of this study are somewhat significant, not only for verifying biological effects of homeopathic doses but for showing that these medicines have some type of radiational effect through glass. Some types of unconventional approaches to homeopathy have been developed over the past decades in which pupil reflex, pulse, muscle strength, and skin conductance have been changed as the result of simply holding on to a bottle of an individually indicated homeopathic medicine.[12]

Although intriguing, such studies may not reflect external reality; these studies have not yet met scientific standards. If bottles are radiating something, other questions and problems arise:

- Action-at-a-distance is a common phenomenon in science. If bottles containing homeopathic remedies are sending out waves or energy, the flow should be measurable directly as waves or energy, independent of any healing effect. No such phenomena have been detected.
- Why doesn't the remedy run down or run out? With healing power leaving all the time, something in the bottle should be decreasing, but homeopaths claim that the remedies do not weaken with time.
- If water clusters are the active component, they must somehow act remotely since they are trapped in the bottle.
- Might not different remedies affect each other on the shelf at home or in stores, or in the kits that both professional and self-prescribers use, since they are all irradiating each other?

Some homeopaths report sending the healing power of a remedy to a patient by holding the remedy near the telephone when the patient is on the other end of the line. Alternatively, if the homeopath has a photograph of or a hair from the patient, the remedy is placed near these objects and the patient receives the healing effect of the remedy. Using such "witnesses" for the patient is reminiscent of voodoo.

Sugar pills apparently can be medicated psychically. Homeopath John Boulderstone tries to experience the symptoms of his patients during case taking. He then thinks of a remedy and senses whether his experience of his patient's symptoms changes; if they lessen, he knows the remedy is the right one. He then gives a plain virgin sugar pill to the patient along with his "understanding" as to what the remedy needs to be.[13]

A number of homeopaths use no physical remedies at all, believing that it is just as effective to write the name and potency of the prescription on a piece of paper and have the patient carry the paper, preferably on the left side of the body.[14] What is the evidence that this procedure works? Eileen Nauman, a proponent of this method, has this to say: "Because I'm Native American and we don't have the word 'why' in our language, I don't bother with the need to know why paper remedies work; I only know that they do."[15]

Some homeopaths have no remedies or names on papers. They consult with their patient by phone and then send the healing effects of the remedy by phone just using their minds.[16] Another indication that physical remedies are not needed is that some people experience their symptoms starting to disappear before they take their remedy.[17]

Jacques Benveniste uses technology to transmit remedies. Skeptic Robert Park reports:

> Benveniste . . . claims to have discovered that the information is stored in the water in the form of electromagnetic waves that can be picked up by a coil surrounding the water. The information, according to Benveniste, can be stored in a computer and transmitted over the Internet to activate water anywhere in the world.[18]

A few homeopaths do not need any help; they use no remedies, no paper and pencil, no phones or computers. Once they have taken the case and determined the needed remedy, they send it telepathically to the patient, wherever he or she may be.

Even the wrong remedy can work. Homeopath Jennifer Smith reviewed some of her old allergy and asthma cases and came to an interesting conclusion:

As I went back through my patient charts, had I not known better, I would
have thought I was on drugs during the time I had prescribed remedies for
those cases. "How could anyone trained in homeopathy come up with that
remedy for that case?" I asked myself time and again as I reviewed the
cases. It was somewhat depressing to read those cases, but I had to chalk
it up as a learning experience. In spite of feeling that way, 76 percent of
the patients showed marked improvement. This proved to me that care
and compassion definitely play a role in homeopathy.[19]

All of these techniques can have internal reality for the practitioners;
the methods can feel as if they are working. However, if it does not matter
whether the remedy is the "right" one, or how it is taken, or even whether
it is taken at all, this further supports the hypothesis that the remedies themselves are not part of the healing process.

UNORTHODOX PROVINGS

Not only do patients not need to take a remedy in order to be cured by it; provers
also need not take the remedy to prove it. In this regard, Rajan Sankaran comments, "The most characteristic symptoms of the drug was [sic] produced in a
woman (seminar participant) who had not taken the proving dose!"[20]

Another claim is that family members who are not participating in
provings are still influenced by the remedy. "Several other children, who
did not have contact with the remedy whose parents were provers, also had
strong new symptoms consistent with the remedy."[21]

Some entire provings are conducted in which *nobody* takes the remedy. In
trituration provings, the provers make the remedy by the trituration process.
The belief is that the participants will get the symptoms as if they had taken the
remedy. In *dream provings*, the remedy is placed under the prover's pillow; it
is then assumed that the prover's dreams are influenced by the remedy.[22]

In *paper provings*, the name of the remedy is written on a piece of
paper and kept close to the body day and night. Reportedly, the symptoms
parallel those in which the remedy is actually taken.[23] In *online provings*, a
homeopath mentally transmits a substance "with the intention that all
present in her chat room will 'receive' this substance."[24] The participants
then report their symptoms.

In *meditative provings*, a prover simply meditates about the remedy.
The following is the introduction to a meditative proving of Apis mellifica,
a bee remedy:

Some Paracelsan/Steinerian thoughts about Apis derived-received while observing bees working clover flowers in a field near Bristol most of the day on Sunday 7 July 1996. The basic ideas were obtained in the field and then extended, organized and fleshed-out through further contemplation as I remained under the influence of the experience for several days. In essence the method is to be with the remedy for some time letting it play in the mind and absorbing its properties, qualities and characteristics, remaining open and receptive to its presence while observing it neutrally and carefully.[25]

Meditation is not a blind process. It is not surprising that the meditation on bees would result in the following main themes:

- Self versus the group, devotion, loyalty, loss of identity, identity only through the group and social conditioning, political structures, communes, etc.
- The domination through very strong attractions to daylight, continuous activity, travel, bright colors, scents, sweetness, etc.
- The theme of burrowing, chambers, tunneling, compartments, and dwellings.[26]

Sometimes homeopaths find support for provings symptoms in strange places. The fact that the date for the proving of Thiosinamine was delayed was believed to indicate that the remedy includes themes of waiting patiently and wasted time.[27]

How do homeopaths explain provings symptoms in people who do not take the remedy? Misha Norland explains, "The psychic field effect of group proving is such that it is not possible for susceptible persons to absent themselves."[28] Rajan Sankaran speaks of "communal consciousness"; others talk about the "psychic field effect" and the "collective unconscious." An alternative explanation is that the remedies cause no symptoms and all people are susceptible to life's vagaries, so of course nonprovers will have some symptoms similar to those of the provers. If the nonparticipants know what is being proved or even just see or hear about the symptoms of those taking the remedy, they may expect and therefore develop similar symptoms.

Some homeopaths express skepticism about these proving issues. Vithoulkas argues:

When, in a proving, you have the same or similar symptoms with placebo as with the remedy, the logical conclusion should be that such symptoms do not belong to the remedy but rather to environmental, circumstantial, or psychological conditions (hysteria, suggestion, anxiety, etc.) but surely not to the remedy! It is most regrettable that somebody managed to persuade novices in homeopathy that placebo symptoms can belong to the proving of the remedy through a metaphysical medium which is the communal consciousness![29]

If one is testing the effects of ingesting the remedy, people who do not take the remedy in provings should be serving as controls; any symptoms they get which the provers also get should not be counted; that is the whole point of having a control group and the way to determine if the remedies *cause* the symptoms.

FAMILY MATTERS

Homeopaths strive to find the simillimum. If a case seems not to point to a single remedy, one solution is to obtain symptoms of family members and other relatives, combine these with the patient's own symptoms, and prescribe a remedy accordingly. This way, "One can construct a sharper image of the remedy required."[30] Here is an example. "Schadde related the case of a child whose painful constipation was mirroring the mother's resistance to falling in love outside of her marriage. After a consultation, the mother embraced the 'shadow' feelings of guilt about her infatuation, and after a dose of Ignatia, the child released her stool."[31] Some homeopaths use events during pregnancy or even events in the parents' lives before conception to select the remedy for a child.[32] Even more extreme is the belief that treating parents before conception can prevent physical and mental abnormalities in children.[33] While it is true that the more symptoms one has, the better is the chance that a single remedy will stand out, it is not at all obvious that using symptoms from people other than the patient will help cure the patient. Classical homeopathy is supposed to treat the whole person, not two or three people as one.

SYNCHRONOUS PHENOMENA

Some homeopaths see remarkable coincidences associated with provings. Jeremy Sherr comments:

It is not entirely surprising that during the proving a great number of strangely synchronous events occur which are strongly related to the proving substance. For instance on the first day of the Neon proving the most sensitive prover woke to find that someone had dumped some old neon lights in her garden. The week I began the proving of Hydrogen two scientists announced that they had achieved nuclear fusion at room temperature [cold fusion]. Three months later, just as the proving was over, the experiment was declared false and invalid. However about three years later, on the day that I published the proving, a newspaper article appeared in which a repeat claim was once again announced. During the proving of Diamond, South Africa held its first general election and several television programs on diamonds were screened, both in the UK and America. Again these phenomena are reported by other proving organizers.[34]

Others have noted astrological correlations, such as Pluto being in Sagittarius when Plutonium was proven.

Statisticians would not find such correlations remarkable. In the year of the Diamond proving or in *any* year, it is not difficult to find some event in the world related to diamonds, for example, changes in their market price, new industrial or scientific uses for diamonds, a new deposit containing diamonds, or a new record-size diamond, or a new way to make diamonds, or countries that mine diamonds, or people who cut or market diamonds, or museums that display famous diamonds. Similarly in any year, something can be found relating to plutonium: the weapons in which it is used, disposal of plutonium waste, use of plutonium in reactors to make electricity, or something scientific or astrological about the planet Pluto. The phenomena cited by Sherr may be close in time, but the implication that they are somehow related is unlikely.

PALEONTOLOGY

Nancy Herrick expresses the unusual belief that remedy provings could assist paleontologists. She discusses a proving of a remedy derived from a fossilized Maiasaura bone. Paleontologists know nothing about the sexual behavior of the dinosaur Maiasaura, but Herrick speculates that "the proving may give us further insight" into their sexual behavior since four dreams of the provers concerned decadent sexuality.[35] That remedies cause dreams or any other symptoms is far from proven, but it is a big leap of faith to assume that the content of the dreams has anything to do with the behavior of the source of the remedy. What if provers of a sandstone remedy had the same type of dream? Should we then conclude that sandstone has wild and decadent sexual behavior? What if a prover of horse bones dreamed that he could breathe water with no ill effects; are we to infer that horses are amphibious?

MUSIC REMEDIES

Music can be stimulating or soothing and thus play a general role in certain kinds of healing and well-being, but some homeopaths see more specific healing power in music. J. P. Jansen has conducted music provings. For instance, volunteers listened to a movement from a Mahler symphony. During and immediately afterward, they wrote down all their thoughts, feelings, and physical symptoms. Jansen then found a remarkable parallel between Mahler's life and the recorded symptoms, including piercing pain in the throat. In addition, Jansen believes that when patients exhibit the symptoms experienced by the music provers, they can be cured by listening to the same music. Others claim to have put the healing power of music (and movies and books) inside potentized remedies.[36]

Rajan Sankaran expressed his conviction that *anything* that heals is related to homeopathy: "I felt that, as music has healing qualities, it must be related to Homeopathy."[37] Like Jansen, he has conducted music provings and included provers' recalled memories as symptoms. Unlike Jansen, Sankaran did not relate the feelings and memories to those of the composer. In fact, the provers' memories and feelings revealed no consistent content. However, Sankaran found consistency in the depth and intensity of the feelings and remembered situations, and he found that the depth and intensity was different for different music. For example, a particular piece of music evoked feelings of warmth and love in an Indian proving and sadness and aloneness in a Western proving. Sankaran perceived a common theme of warmth or loss of warmth. Apparently, if one does not find common symptoms, opposite symptoms can be interpreted to represent a common theme. With such abstract and subjective approaches, it is easy to find commonality between *any* data sets.

On occasion Sankaran prescribes music instead of remedies, and tapes of "proven" music are sold by his publisher. In such cases, there are no material remedies, no concept of minimum dose, and no potentization. Music can be therapeutic, but is it homeopathy?

AUTOMOBILE FIRST AID

Even automobiles can ostensibly benefit from homeopathic care. A well-known practitioner, Eileen Nauman, reported that a friend of hers fixed a car homeopathically. The friend's son was having car problems. Since the problems seemed to be electrical, the young man's father suggested writing "Electricitas 200C" on a piece of paper and placing the paper near the engine. Doing this enabled the car to complete a trip from California to the East Coast.[38]

SOME INTERESTING REMEDIES

Homeopathy has some remedies that even before potentization are especially difficult to understand in a scientific context (table 13.1). One category is remedies made from materials one would not think of as medicinal, such as the Berlin wall, Braille paper, stainless steel, newsprint, granite, polyurethane, xenon, Stonehenge, whole wheat bread, New York City,[39] dog's ear wax, tears from a weeping young girl, and Powerbook 165 (a computer).

Water and alcohol, the workhorse solvents used in the preparation of homeopathic remedies, are both considered to be remedies in their own right. Waters from different sources (springs, lakes, and rivers) are considered distinct remedies. Ice (Aqua crystalisata) is considered a remedy distinct from the water remedies despite the fact that the ice melts to water at the very beginning of the process of making the remedy.

Table 13.1. Some Remedies That Especially Challenge Known Science	
Name	**Ingredient(s) if not apparent from name**
Aqua . . .	Water (roughly twenty different remedies from different water sources)
Aqua crystalisata	Ice
Snow flake	
Computer terminal rays	
Colored light: red, orange, yellow, green, turquoise, indigo, violet, pink, magenta, and "spectrum"	
Ignis alcoholis	Burning alcohol
Luna	Moonlight
Lunar eclipse	Eclipsed moonlight
Magnetis poli ambo	Both poles, or the side of a bar magnet
Magnetis polus arcticus	North pole of a magnet
Magnetis polus australis	South pole of a magnet
Positronium	Antimatter
Sol britannic	Sunlight
Solar eclipse ray	
Ultrasound—3.5 megahertz	
Vacuum	
Ventus	Wind
X-rays	

The imponderable remedies are difficult for scientists to understand. For colored light remedies,[40] the initial tincture is made by exposing water or alcohol in a clear glass container to the particular color of light; technical details are not given. Sol is a sunlight remedy: "Saccharum lactis is exposed to concentrated sun's rays and stirred with a glass rod till saturated."[41] No information is given about how one knows when the lactose is saturated, and it is curious that direct sunlight is believed by most homeopaths to deactivate any homeopathic remedy. That exposing water, alcohol, or lactose to moonlight should make a useful remedy (Luna) is hard for a scientist to accept; to claim that light from an eclipsed moon makes a different remedy (Lunar eclipse) is even harder to fathom.

Why are these remedies difficult for a scientist to accept? When visible light from any source shines through water or alcohol, the vast majority of it passes on through; that is what makes water and alcohol clear liquids. What little energy is absorbed will serve only to make the liquid a little warmer. The temperature rise itself will be affected much more by the surrounding air temperature, the infrared component of the light, and the light's overall brightness than by the visible color or particular source of the light.

If light did have a lasting impact on the water, the initial intentional illumination would probably not be dominant. Most water would have been exposed to much more light before its use to make a remedy than during the intentional exposure, especially if the water came from a reservoir, lake, or stream. Even most well water was once in the atmosphere and so exposed to bright sunlight for a long time. High temperatures are said to deactivate homeopathic remedies; thus if distilled water (distillation involves boiling) is used, its previous history should not matter. However, in the subsequent dilutions, unless the dilutions were done in total darkness, the water would again be exposed to light. When the remedy is stored or used, it is again exposed to light. Light remedies typically come in amber glass bottles that block only some light. How is the remedy to know that it was only the one brief intentional illumination that determined its healing effects?

Most light-based remedies should either have no curative power or be nearly identical because they would be mixtures of the curative powers of all visible colors. Thus it seems unlikely that such remedies would be very useful, a view shared by a few homeopaths.

Much the same can be said about remedies based on electricity (electrons), electric and magnetic fields, x-rays, and gamma radiation. Most of these are traditional remedies, having been in use for over one hundred years. During the exposure, these types of influences can raise the temperature very slightly, give the molecules a preferred orientation, and ionize the molecules causing some structural rearrangement. None of these phenomena has any lasting effect on the exposed water; the water returns to its pre-exposure condition, except for the possible slight temperature rise, within a fraction of a second after the exposure ends.

All of these effects permeate our world. Electric and magnetic fields, x-rays, and gamma radiation are part of our natural environment and penetrate through amber bottles with no difficulty. Thus the liquid will have been exposed before the remedy is made, and the liquid or pellet remedy will continue to be exposed continuously until a patient takes it. Which of all these exposures is the remedy supposed to represent?

Magnetic remedies have all the above problems with an added internal contradiction. There are three distinct magnetic remedies—a north pole remedy, a south pole remedy, and a combination pole remedy. They have different symptoms and therein lies the problem. When a magnet is held close to a container of water or alcohol to turn it into a remedy, the only difference between using the north or south pole is the direction of the magnetic field. Field direction makes no difference for a homogeneous material like liquid water or alcohol, and even if field direction did matter, bringing a north pole up to the left side of a bottle results in the same field direction as bringing a south pole up to the right side of the bottle (figure 13.1). Thus it should make no difference at all which pole is used.[42]

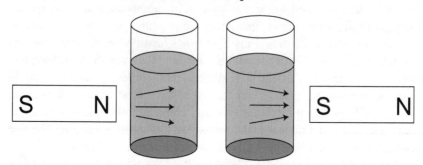

Figure 13.1. Why north pole and south pole homeopathic remedies should be indistinguishable. The arrows represent the direction of the magnetic field.

Hahnemann knew much less about the science of magnets than we do today. Given today's knowledge, the fact that north and south pole remedies were reported by Hahnemann and his contemporaries as inducing different symptoms calls into question the symptoms they reported for all remedies.

There is no conventional scientific reason why any of these imponderable remedies should have any healing effect or why any of them should be distinguishable from any other or, in fact, from plain water or plain sugar.

The ultimate imponderable remedy is a relatively new one made from a vacuum. Nuala Eising reports:

> On January 2nd, 1999, I procured a vacuum pump of the type generally used to take the air out of wine bottles. I obtained an unused, brown 500 mL bottle with an opening that would fit the vacuum pump. I washed the bottle numerous times in pure alcohol. I put 20 mL of pure alcohol into the bottle, and then used the pump to create a vacuum. I left the alcohol in the bottle for seven hours, checking at frequent intervals to ensure that the vacuum was maintained. I also succussed the bottle every hour (40 succussions) so as to ensure that the alcohol was affected by the vacuum. After this, I opened the bottle and took three drops of alcohol and added it to 297 drops of un-vacuumed, pure alcohol. I succussed the mixture and got the 1C potency. I continued in this manner until I had developed the 30C potency.[43]

That this remedy should have any effects is almost inconceivable to a scientist. A vacuum is empty space, void of all molecules, atoms and electrons. Alcohol molecules are not altered in a vacuum. If alcohol and a vacuum are mixed, all one can get is alcohol. A more technical criticism is that there cannot be a vacuum over liquid alcohol at room temperature; the alcohol will evaporate until it reaches what is called its vapor pressure, which is on the order of 5 to 10 percent of atmospheric pressure. If 20 mL of room temperature alcohol were in a true vacuum for a short time, it would all evaporate.

Yet, this remedy is reported to have caused symptoms in a proving. A strong theme was that "people seemed to need to project beyond the material dimension to find a meaning or purpose and to experience the spirit world which existed before the material."[44]

CONVENTIONAL MEDICINE AND LICENSING

Conventional medicine has its own fringe. Some M.D.s treat patients using practices and theories that have only anecdotal support and seem implausible. Many examples of such practices can be found in cancer treatment and prevention.[45] However, conventional medicine and homeopathy treat their fringes differently. Because there is not yet convincing evidence of efficacy, the majority of conventional physicians do not expect fringe treatments to have any value. If there were evidence, the treatment would not be on the fringe but in the mainstream. In contrast, the homeopathic fringe is automatically given credibility by most practicing homeopaths; after all, the fringe practitioners report having some cured cases. A key difference is that conventional medicine generally has different standards for evidence than homeopathy.

This difference exists because most practicing homeopaths are not M.D.s. Unlike M.D.s, most homeopaths practice without a license (legal recognition and regulation by the state) and many practice without certification (evidence of training and competency, needed for licensing). Homeopathy is unregulated or ignored in many states, and where it is regulated, the enforcers have little incentive and no clear guidelines for rejecting fringe practices within homeopathy. Thus, in most states, anyone claiming to be a homeopath can practice homeopathy in any fashion he or she wishes. These loose standards result in a great variety of backgrounds and training and consequently a broad range of views on topics such as what is and is not homeopathy and what constitutes convincing evidence. In contrast, M.D.s have more training in distinguishing between anecdotal and substantial evidence, and since M.D.s are licensed and regulated, they can and do lose their licenses to practice if the efficacy and/or safety of their practice becomes too far removed from proven or accepted practices.

CONCLUSION

There is a full range of reactions to homeopathy's fringe practices. To the unquestioning believers in homeopathy, these practices are just business as usual. Some homeopaths see the apparent success of fringe practices as proof that homeopathy is metaphysical and that science can never understand it.

Some practitioners find the homeopathic fringe exhilarating and liberating. Each individual homeopath is free to try new approaches, and when they appear to work, the practitioner feels empowered. This is the same excitement scientists feel when making a discovery but without the methodological constraints designed to help assure that the conclusion reflects external reality.

Those with active inquiring minds find the fringe a fascinating and exciting challenge to try to explain, but in their excitement they may overlook the important first step of establishing the reality of the claim—that the patients' or provers' changed health was actually *caused* by the remedy.

Some homeopaths find the fringe embarrassing and detrimental to homeopathy; they may secretly wish the fringe would disappear, but publicly ask only that the word *homeopathy* not be applied to fringe practices.

Diehard skeptics also see these fringe practices as business as usual. They find fringe homeopathy no more unbelievable than classical homeopathy with its nonmolecular remedies and absence of any plausible mechanism. They feel that evidence meeting basic scientific standards is lacking in both cases. The fact that many homeopaths uncritically accept the effectiveness of fringe practices adds to the skeptics' conviction that the whole field has no basis in reality.

NOTES

1. Bill Gray, *Homeopathy: Science or Myth?* (Berkeley: North Atlantic Books, 2000), p. 52.

2. Jörg Wichmann, "Defining a Different Tradition for Homeopathy," *Homoeopathic Links* 14, no. 4 (2001): 202–203.

3. Robert Ullman and Judyth Reichenberg-Ullman, *The Patient's Guide to Homeopathic Medicine* (Edmonds, Wash.: Picnic Point Press, 1995), p. 49.

4. D. Quaranto, "Remedies and Rituals," *Simillimum* 13, no. 2 (2000): 67.

5. Luc De Schepper, "LM Potencies: One of the Hidden Treasures of the Sixth Edition of the *Organon*," *British Homeopathic Journal* 88 (1999): 133.

6. Julian Winston, editorial introduction to Magda Aguila, "Undercover: Homeopathy in the Neonatal Unit," *Homeopathy Today* 22, no. 1 (2002): 19.

7. Denise Philpott, "I Didn't Know Homeopathy Could Treat *That!* The Creative Use of Remedies," *Homeopathy Today* 22, no. 2 (2002): 6.

8. Interview with André Saine, *Homoeopathic Links* 14, no. 2 (2001): 122; and P. Wright, "Nature is Generous," summary of a seminar by André Saine, *Simillimum* 13, no. 2 (2000): 99.

9. Richard Moskowitz, *Resonance: The Homeopathic Point of View* (www.Xlibris.com, Xlibris Corporation, 2000), p. 36.

10. Julian Winston, *Homeopathy Digest for July 4, 1996* [online], http://www.homeopathy.plus.com/Homeopathy_List_Archive/1996/04_July/Homeopathy%20Digest%20for%204%20Jul%201996.txt [Aug. 4, 2002]; and Misha Norland, letters to the editor, *Homoeopathic Links* 13, no. 3 (2000).

11. Winston, *Homeopathy Digest*.

12. Dana Ullman, *The Consumer's Guide to Homeopathy* (New York: G. P. Putnam's Sons, 1995), pp. 57–58.

13. John Boulderstone, "The Next Step," *Homeopath*, no. 77 (2000).

14. Eileen Nauman, letters to the editor, *Homoeopathic Links* 13, no. 4 (2000).

15. Ibid.

16. Mahlom Wagner, "Is Homeopathy 'New Science' or 'New Age'?" *Scientific Review of Alternative Medicine* 1, no. 1 (1997): 10.

17. Allan Coniglio, Lyghtforce e-mail list, *Homeopathy Digest* 3, no. 211 (2002), archives online at http://www.lyghtforce.com/HomeoList.

18. Robert Park, *Voodoo Science: The Road from Foolishness to Fraud* (New York: Oxford University Press, 2000), p. 57.

19. Jennifer Smith, "Gifts from Homeopathy," *Simillimum* 13, no. 2 (2000): 15–18.

20. Rajan Sankaran, *The Substance of Homeopathy* (Mumbai, India: Homoeopathic Medical Publishers, 1994), p. 5.

21. Nancy Herrick, *Animal Mind, Human Voices: Provings of Eight New Animal Remedies* (Nevada City, Calif.: Hahnemann Clinic Publishing, 1998), p. xiv.

22. Peter Konig and Uta Santl-Konig, "Berberis, Rhododendron, Convallaria: From Dream Essences to Essential Remedies" [online], http://www.lyghtforce.com/HomeopathyOnline/text/koenig_book.htm [May 26, 2002].

23. Nauman.

24. Online proving conducted Nov. 4, 2002, by the Online Homeopathic Resource (www.olne.net). The quotation is from e-mail received Oct. 26, 2002, from support@olne.net announcing the event.

25. Peter Morrell, "Apis Mellifica: A Paracelsan Meditative Proving" [online], http://homeoint.org/morrell/articles/pm_apis.htm [May 26, 2002].

26. Ibid., with minor edits.

27. T. Grinney, "Proving of Thiosinamine: Author's Reply," letter to the editor, *British Homeopathic Journal* 90, no. 3 (2001): 173.

28. Misha Norland, "A Proving of Falcon Blood and Feather" [online], http://www. hominf.org/falc/falcfr.htm [Nov. 30, 2002].

29. George Vithoulkas, "A Proving of Thiosinamine," letter to the editor, *British Homeopathic Journal* 90, no. 3 (2001): 172.

30. S. Goldsmith, "Homeopathic Family Diagnosis: The Fifth Dimension," *Journal of the American Institute of Homeopathy* 93, no. 3 (2000), p. 116.

31. Tina Quirk, "From Beryllium to Zingiber: Report on a Presentation by Anne Schadde, April 5–6, 2002, New York," *Homeopathy Today* 22, no. 9 (2002): 34–35.

32. Luc De Schepper, *Hahnemann Revisited* (Santa Fe: Full of Life Publishing, 2001), pp. 202–204; and Melanie Chimes, "Severe Behavioral and Emotional Problems in Children," *Homeopathy Today* 22, no. 9 (2002):14–16.

33. Luc De Schepper, p. 362.

34. Jeremy Sherr, *The Dynamics and Methodology of Homeopathic Provings* (Malvern, U.K.: Dynamis Books, 1995), pp. 33–34.

35. Nancy Herrick, p. 270.

36. Paul Herscu, *Provings Volume, with a Proving of Alcoholus* (Amherst, Mass.: New England School of Homeopathy Press, 2002), p. 75.

37. Sankaran, p. 293.

38. Nauman.

39. Herscu, p. 80.

40. Ambika Wauters, *Homeopathic Color Remedies* (Freedom, Calif.: Crossing Press, 1999). Light-based remedies are used but not officially recognized in the United States. They are not included in the HPUS.

41. John Henry Clarke, *A Dictionary of Practical Materia Medica*, vol. 3 (1902; reprint, New Delhi: B. Jain Publishers, 2000), p. 1202.

42. The preparation of the third magnetic remedy starts with exposure "to the influence of the entire magnet." Clarke, vol. 2, p. 379.

43. Nuala Eising, *Vacuum: The Proving* (Galway, Ireland: Burren School of Homeopathy, 2000), p. 3.

44. Ibid., p. 6.

45. "A Special Message for Cancer Patients Seeking 'Alternative' Treatments" [online], http://www.quackwatch.com/00AboutQuackwatch/altseek.html [Nov. 30, 2002].

14. *The Mechanisms of Misperception*

Homeopathy thrives today in many different nations with diverse cultures, as it has for nearly two centuries. The primary reason is simple: It works, in the sense that most patients are better after treatment. Almost all the patients and practitioners in all these countries over all these years have believed that the remedies caused the improvement in health, yet the scientific evidence on the remedies being active is weak and theoretical problems and contradictions abound. Overall, it seems likely that the remedies are not an active part of the health benefits. Is it possible that so many patients and practitioners in so many places over such a long time have been wrong about the role of the remedies?

The possibility of such a misperception is not entirely unrecognized by those close to and within homeopathy. Wayne Jonas, former director of the National Institute of Health's Office of Alternative Medicine, says, "The capacity of humans to fool themselves by making claims of truth, postulating unfounded explanations, and denying the reality of observations they cannot explain is endless. Science has emerged as one of the few truly powerful approaches for mitigating this self-delusionary capacity."[1] Author Julian Winston and homeopath Chris Kurz even worry that homeopaths do not always accurately perceive patients' health.

> There are cases presented by internationally acclaimed speakers where those present see no cure happening—contrary to what the author/speaker

says. We may want to believe that cure *is* happening and so we may give them the benefit of the doubt; it's part of our collective "delusion" and an aspect of our practices that we should carefully monitor.[2]

How could so many people have misconstrued the evidence for so long? This chapter explores and attempts to explain the belief in remedies that probably do not work and summarizes key points from the previous chapters.

SUMMARY OF EVIDENCE THAT MOST HOMEOPATHIC REMEDIES ARE INACTIVE

The strongest direct evidence for the inactivity of remedies is the fact that in clinical trials designed to measure the effect of the remedies themselves, the statistical significance and the clinical significance both seem to approach zero as the methodological quality approaches contemporary scientific standards. The number of symptoms attributable to the remedies in provings also approaches zero as methodological quality approaches contemporary scientific standards. Important indirect evidence is the fact that all the methods of selecting the remedy seem to work about equally well, as do all the ways of taking the remedy, including not taking it or taking the wrong remedy.

This section summarizes all the evidence and arguments that support the inactivity of homeopathic remedies by noting the contradictions and unsolved problems that no longer exist if the remedies are inactive.

Theory:

- Now we can understand why homeopaths believe that *everything* is a potential remedy—everything they have tried would appear equally effective if the healing is independent of the remedy, including inert substances such as water, xenon, and snowflakes.
- Imponderable remedies that have no atoms to start with would no longer be doubly inexplicable.
- The claim that nonmolecular remedies are at least as effective as the less dilute remedies would make sense if the healing is not due to the remedies.
- It would no longer be necessary to explain why the water memory of a substance would be more effective then the substance itself.
- The claim that remedies are equally effective for the same ailments

in reptiles, birds, and mammals would not need justification if there were no longer any pretense of a direct biochemical mechanism.

- An explanation would no longer be needed for how, in tautopathy, the remedy fights the side effects of conventional drugs but not their intended primary action.
- No explanation would be needed for how a remedy knows to represent only the intended initial medicinal ingredient and not all the contaminants that enter at every stage of the process (Appendix 4).
- An explanation would no longer be needed for exactly why the same pill can induce and cure the same symptoms (in provings and with patients, respectively).

Remedies:

- The details of succussion would no longer matter—pounding the bottle on a leather book, or shaking it, or stirring it would all have the same noneffect.
- The debate over Hahnemannian versus Korsakovian methods (Appendix 1) for making remedies would be unnecessary; they would appear to be equally effective because neither would affect the remedies.
- No explanation would be needed for why triturated remedies are just as effective (or ineffective) as succussed remedies even though the processes are very different.
- Expanding the supply of a remedy by grafting or plussing would indeed yield equally "active" remedies.
- Remedies made by placing water or unmedicated pellets on paper with a remedy's name written on it would be as active as any others.

Provings:

If the remedies themselves do not cause the symptoms in (nontoxic) provings, the symptoms come from the natural ups and downs of health, expectations and imagination, and supervisor prodding and interpretation. Then all the following issues would be resolved:

- The fact that provings with the highest methodological quality tend to produce the fewest symptoms attributable to the remedies would make sense since the other causes of symptoms are accounted for and excluded.
- Theories of the collective unconscious, communal consciousness,

and the psychic field effect would no longer be needed to explain why people who do not take the remedy get some of the same symptoms as those who do in provings; the absence of remedies and the remedies would be equally "active."

- The fact that provings in which no one takes the remedy (dream, trituration, and meditative provings) seem to work as well as normal provings would be explained.
- The theory that each prover "brings out" different symptoms of the remedy due to the provers' differing sensitivities would no longer be needed; provers would get different symptoms because people's natural health problems are different, as are their dreams, fears, likes, and dislikes.
- That the same remedy can cause opposite symptoms (for example, constipation and diarrhea) would no longer need explanation. One would nearly always find some diarrhea and constipation in any group of people over a period of time, and such symptoms could easily be interpreted as unusual in some sense so that they could be interpreted as having been caused by the remedy.
- Similarly, asymmetric symptoms, such as pain in only the right leg, hand, or foot and not the left, would no longer need to be reconciled with science, in which no ingested substance has ever been known to have an inherently asymmetric impact on symmetric parts of the body.
- There would now be an explanation for why overproved remedies have similar symptom pictures; if the symptoms come from the normal vicissitudes of health, the distributions should look similar when the number of symptoms is large.

Selecting the Simillimum and the Potency:

- The fact that the aches, pains, and diseases that cause a patient to seek medical help are the least important symptoms when a homeopath selects the remedy would no longer seem so strange; none of the symptoms would be critical for selecting the remedy because the particular remedy does not matter.
- If the remedies are not part of the cure, it would make sense that the dozens of ways for selecting remedies would all seem to work, despite the fact that different remedies are usually selected.
- Similarly, it would make sense that some homeopaths have found the "wrong" remedy to be as effective as the "right" remedy.

- The claim that any potency will do would make sense.
- The weakness of the Law of Similars would not undermine homeopathy.

Storing and Taking Remedies:

- The amount of remedy taken at any one time would not matter—one pill or two hundred and fifty would have the same healing effect if the pills themselves are not active, aside from a possible sugar "high."
- Pills would appear to have unlimited shelf life if the pills are not part of the healing.
- The fact that dose frequencies ranging from one remedy every thirty seconds to one every year or more both seem to be effective would be no surprise.
- The claims of complete safety and no side effects would make sense if nothing is there but the carrier—usually a small amount of sugar.
- All intake modes (oral, topical, injected, etc.) would appear to be equally effective.
- All the unusual ways of taking remedies—touching, sniffing, putting in one's bath water, just carrying the bottle, just carrying a piece of paper with the name written on it, and telephone and psychic transmission—would no longer need explanations for how the healing power is transferred to the patient.
- People are admonished not to eat or drink within fifteen minutes of taking a remedy, but animals are usually given their remedies by mixing them with their food or water. If remedies are inactive, it would be clear why these contradictory procedures appear equally effective.
- The huge array of environmental conditions that sometimes deactivate stored remedies and the huge array of patient actions that sometimes antidote the effect of a remedy after it is taken, and the disagreements among homeopaths concerning these factors no longer need explanation: Sometimes patients improve and sometimes they do not after taking a remedy that was inactive to begin with.

Patients' Response to Remedies:

- All the retroactive unprovable explanations such as aggravations and Hering's Laws for why patients do not just get well would no longer be needed.
- Homeopathic success rate with patients apparently has not improved

over two hundred years despite the huge increase in the number of remedies and computer power to help select the simillimum. This fact would be no surprise if the remedy is not the cause of the cures.

- It is hard to reconcile the claimed success of homeopathy with animals, babies, and plants[3] with the claimed importance of mental and emotional symptoms, and the importance of the patient's own words in describing symptoms, unless the remedies are inactive.

Clinical Trials:

- The fact that the higher-quality clinical trials have smaller statistical and clinical significance would be expected if the remedies are ineffective since all other factors are controlled.

Laboratory Research:

- All the elusive and unproven models for the active ingredient in non-molecular remedies would no longer be needed—the water in 30C remedies does not have memory. It is just water.
- All the contradictions between the water cluster model and homeopathic practice would be eliminated.
- It would no longer be frustrating that no laboratory procedure can distinguish high-potency remedies from one another—they are not different from one another.

It cannot be overemphasized that homeopathy still works even if the remedies do not. Not only do patients get better, but homeopathy is the cause of much of this improvement.

WHY REMEDIES APPEAR TO BE RESPONSIBLE

There are four significant reasons why homeopathic remedies are given credit for changes in the patient's health:

1. Homeopathy often does help even if the remedies are not the cause.
2. Correlation seems like causation.
3. Dosage protocol creates the appearance of cause.
4. Getting worse is often counted as getting better.

Benefits of Homeopathy

Homeopathy's reputation for success stems primarily from the fact that many of its patients *are* improved after treatment. As explained in chapter 8, there are many possible reasons for improved health other than an active remedy.

- Unassisted natural healing (especially applicable to acute conditions)—the patient would have recovered just as quickly with no treatment.
- The spaghetti effect—real biochemical or physical healing caused by an as yet unrecognized factor in the patient's life.
- Statistical healing or regression to the mean—the tendency to seek help when conditions are near their worst means that, on average, the patient is more likely to feel better than worse after taking the remedy.
- Nonhomeopathic treatments, previous or concurrent. Some homeopaths recommend concurrent nonhomeopathic treatments.
- The cessation of uncomfortable, painful, or harmful treatments, conventional or alternative. Homeopaths often recommend such cessation.
- Healthier lifestyles, often urged by the homeopath (in part, ostensibly so that the homeopathic remedy can work).
- The placebo response—the expectation of getting better helps the patient get better by activating his or her internal pharmacy.
- The psychological benefits of consultations with a truly caring, nonjudgmental, and patient caregiver.

Confusion of Correlation with Cause

The primary reason that makes it seem like the remedy caused the cure is the human tendency to confuse correlation with cause. We just assume that the last thing that happened must have been the cause. Since homeopaths are always monitoring the patient and prescribing more doses or different potencies or different remedies, especially when the patient is not doing well, the last thing that the patient did before feeling better is often taking a remedy.

Dosage Protocol

As a result of an article by Karl Sabbagh based on an idea proposed by Emil Freireic,[4] the term *fringe medicine* has come to have a specific meaning. By definition, the key elements of fringe medicine are (1) a treatment that does nothing chemically or physically and consequently cannot help or hurt, and (2) a dosing protocol in which the treatment is given if the patient is getting worse and stopped if the patient is getting better.

When these fringe medicine guidelines are applied to human conditions that have variations in symptom intensity, which most conditions do, then any improvement at all will appear to have been caused by the treatment. The patient is to be treated when feeling worse, which is the usual situation in practice. If the patient continues to get worse, this does not indicate the treatment is ineffective but just that the treatment needs to be continued or increased. If the patient stops getting worse, this "proves" the treatment is working; the treatment is continued. If the patient starts getting better, this also "proves" the treatment works. If the patient dies, the treatment is not to blame; the patient did not seek help early enough.

When the patient starts getting better, the treatment is to be stopped. If the patient continues to get better, then "obviously" the treatment is responsible. If the patient's health stays the same or declines after the treatment is stopped, this also "proves" the treatment works—its cessation is why the patient did not continue to improve; the treatment is then resumed.

These procedures of treating when the patient is worsening or stagnant and stopping treatments when the patient is improving provide plausible-sounding explanations for all outcomes—explanations that seem to support the treatment as the cause. Fringe medicine even "works" for diseases for which the overall trend is downward, since the variations in symptoms will still give the appearance of success, albeit temporary. There is rarely fraud in fringe medicine, just understandable self-deception.

Homeopathy's usual dosing protocol fits this fringe model. Patients are often told to take remedies when they feel bad and to stop taking them as soon as they start feeling better.[5] Thus the remedies often *appear* to be the cause of the patient's changes even if the remedies are inactive. This is not to say that homeopathy as a whole is fringe medicine since most of homeopathy's healing mechanisms are effective.

Getting Worse Perceived as Getting Better

Contributing to the feeling that the remedy was the cause is the fact that in homeopathy the remedies are interpreted as being the cause of nearly everything that happens to the patient. If a patient gets worse after taking conventional medicine, the conclusion is that the medicine did not help. However, if a homeopathic patient gets worse, homeopaths often conclude that the remedy caused the worsening and that the worsening is an important part of getting better (aggravations and Hering's Laws). Thus homeopaths claim credit for a much bigger piece of the possible outcome pie, enhancing the impression that their remedies are working.

MISUNDERSTANDING OF SCIENCE CONTRIBUTES TO MISPERCEPTION

How could homeopaths believe so deeply that their remedies cure in face of evidence that they do not? Many factors contribute, but the chief underlying problem is a misunderstanding of science.

Lack of Distinction Between External Reality and Internal Reality

Some people pay little attention to the difference between internal and external reality. For them, there is only one reality, and it is internal. They dismiss what scientists state as irrelevant and unnecessary. They might say, "I know homeopathy works, so there must be something wrong with the scientific tests."

Interpreting internal as external reality ignores all that has been learned about how easy it is to fool ourselves; it ignores how we progressed from the superstitious Dark Ages and how we have come to have our culture and its creature comforts, such as cell phones and jet planes. All of technology is based on the existence of an external reality, and science is the best tool for revealing this reality.

Excessive Faith in Cases

Successful homeopathic cases are improvements in health perceived to be caused by remedies. Homeopaths tend to have strong faith in cases as evidence of the external reality of remedy efficacy. This faith can be traced largely to Hahnemann's reliance on his own cases and to homeopaths' devout belief in Hahnemann. The dangers of depending on cured cases are not understood by most patients or homeopaths. Conventional medicine also is sometimes too reliant on cases. Marcia Angell, M.D., and Jerome Kassirer, M.D., concede: "Of course, many treatments used in conventional medicine have not been rigorously tested, either, but the scientific commu-

nity generally acknowledges that this is a failing that needs to be reme-
died."[6] Homeopaths, in contrast, tend to see such testing as unnecessary.

Patient Satisfaction

Homeopaths see so many satisfied patients that it is natural for them to
interpret this satisfaction as meaning that the remedies work. Clearly something is happening that the patients like; patients feel better because homeopathy as an overall approach usually improves health, and even if it does
not, they like the process. However, the existence of satisfied patients is not
scientific evidence that the remedy is the cause, as is clear from the high
patient satisfaction with so many proven quack and sham health practices
over the last one hundred and fifty years.[7]

Mistrust of Clinical Trials

Testing the efficacy of homeopathic remedies can be more difficult than
testing conventional medicines, but it still can be done. For many
researchers, the challenge of designing and executing difficult projects provides much of the motivation and excitement of being a scientist. The challenges of individualizing of the remedies, of follow-up consultations with
changes in remedy, and of including general quality of life outcomes can
all be met. The research may be complex and expensive, but it is possible.
Homeopaths' inclination to distrust clinical trials may be related to an emotional reaction to trials that do not support homeopathy, and to the fact that
some trials have not had competent input from homeopaths, resulting in
unrealistic homeopathic treatment.

How *Is Not Needed to Determine* Whether

Many homeopaths do not trust the results of clinical trials conducted by non-
homeopath scientists because they realize most scientists cannot understand
how nonmolecular remedies could possibly work. These homeopaths may
not appreciate the fact that science need not have any idea *how* homeopathic
remedies work in order to determine *whether* the remedies work. While it is
true that most scientists are skeptical concerning nonmolecular remedies,
the whole double-blind placebo-controlled random-assignment procedure is
designed to determine *whether* a medicine or other procedure is effective;
no knowledge or opinion of *how* a medicine might work is involved.

Lack of Appreciation for Falsifiable Theories

Homeopaths are comfortable with homeopathic theory because it seems to have a plausible explanation for everything. Every outcome can be made to fit the theory. Thus the theory can never be proven wrong; it is not falsifiable. In addition, most of the individual concepts in homeopathic theory are unmeasurable—they are described vaguely, are defined circularly, or are overtly metaphysical. Concepts that cannot be measured cannot be verified as having external reality.

Homeopaths' comfort with nonfalsifiable theories is understandable. Falsifiability is a somewhat abstract and unfamiliar concept often unmentioned in our educational systems. Furthermore, the complexity of homeopathic theory makes it difficult to see that the theory is nonfalsifiable. Lack of recognition for the importance of falsifiability facilitates acceptance of unsupportable (untestable) beliefs, which in turn facilitates the misperception of the essential role of the remedies.

What About the Miraculous Cures?

Julian Winston explains why he and other homeopaths believe so strongly in the simillimum: "Every homeopath I've met has seen the *one* remedy *really do it* at least once—and it gives them the knowledge that the abstract goal of curing with the single remedy *is possible*."[8]

When a total cure occurs after a single remedy is given to a patient, the remedy still may have nothing to do with the cure. One or more of the other healing modalities could have been the actual cause. When a homeopath sees and treats a very large number of patients, it is statistically probable that such a miraculous "cure" will occasionally be seen to occur because when the total number of events (cases) is very large, rare events are likely to occur. Flipping a coin five times is unlikely to result in five heads; on average five heads in a row will occur only once in every thirty-two attempts. But if one tries it a hundred times, a few successes are probable just due to the laws of probability.)

Quantum Mechanics, Relativity, and Chaos

Homeopaths tend to look toward the most abstract concepts in contemporary physics for possible explanations of how the remedies might work, including concepts related to relativity, quantum mechanics, and chaos theory. This approach is reasonable; explanations may lie in such theories. In practice, the weakness is that most of those doing the speculation are not experts in these subjects, and their speculations are often an incorrect application of the concepts, however attractive they may seem.

The right way to explore this approach is to obtain the opinions of a few highly reputable experts in these fields. It is also important to understand that homeopathy will not be convincingly explained unless quantitative predictions of a physics theory match quantitative data from homeopathy; that is, the results must be *measurable*. Retrospective analogies between homeopathy and theoretical physics may reinforce an internal reality but are not evidence of external realty.

Science Cannot Yet Explain Homeopathy

Some homeopaths are attracted to the idea that even the most esoteric theories of contemporary science are not advanced enough to explain how homeopathic remedies work, nor does science yet have the instrumentation to measure the active ingredient in remedies. Homeopaths believe that their field is analogous to some others, such as plate tectonics, which were rejected for a long time by mainstream science but ultimately embraced. Indeed, such future acceptance is possible, but most homeopaths may not be aware that the vast majority of ideas that could not be explained by contemporaneous science, when first proposed, turned out to be wrong—they did not describe external reality.

Close-Mindedness and Conspiracy Theories

Most homeopaths are so convinced that their remedies work that the resistance of physicians and scientists is incomprehensible to them. Many homeopaths believe physicians and scientists are either too close-minded to see the "obvious" evidence or are motivated by money. Many homeopaths believe that drug companies and physicians are conspiring to suppress homeopathy because it competes for customers.

Such conspiracy theories seem weak for two reasons. (1) Nonscientists do not realize the extraordinary excitement, fame, and fortune that await the discoverers of radically new phenomena that do not fit into previous scientific knowledge; scientists yearn for such opportunities. True science has no interest in suppressing discoveries. (2) Conspiracies require keeping secrets, and large conspiracies need large numbers of people to keep secrets. People are not good at keeping secrets, and there are many sound reasons not to keep secret knowledge that homeopathic remedies really are biologically active.

The primary reasons for most physicians' skepticism of homeopathy are that many of its claims are contrary to known science, and the experimental evidence that the remedies work is not convincing.

Reliance on Authority

Although Hahnemann's writings are historically significant, they are irrelevant for establishing external reality. If homeopathy were a science, it would not matter what Hahnemann said. He would always get credit for having pioneered the field, but the validity of homeopaths' claims would be determined solely by scientifically valid experiments and observations. External reality is determined by nature and revealed by measurements. Some contemporary homeopaths recognize the problem of reliance on authority: "Quoting 'Masters' is sectarian and no scientist will take us seriously if we really believe that a book written 200 years ago is the measure for our thinking and practice."[9]

Homeopathy Is **Already** *Scientific*

Discussions about using science to determine the external validity of homeopathy sound silly to some homeopaths. Their internal reality is that homeopathy is solidly scientific; Hahnemann said so, and so do most of modern authors and teachers in the field. Many homeopaths think that homeopathy is more scientific than conventional medicine and voice sentiments such as:

> Conventional medicine calls itself scientific, but where are its fixed principles and laws, which are the foundation of any true science?[10]

> The student must master the science—the infallible Laws of Nature upon which it [homeopathy] is founded.[11]

> Homeopathy is scientific medicine; its rules were developed by following the procedures of the scientific method. Homeopathic medications are prepared according to an exact process and prescribed according to the Law of Similars.[12]

Homeopaths appear to believe that science consists of immutable laws and fixed meticulous procedures—a system that is defined and constrained. Card games and sports also have well-defined rules and procedures; this fact does not make them scientific. The essence of science includes none of these characteristics. Science asks questions, is skeptical, gathers data, strives for the simplest and most powerful (predictive) theory, judges theories with data from controlled tests, and does not hesitate to admit that historically important scientists were sometimes wrong. Most important, science is open and eager to change its "laws" in the face of convincing data. Engineers work with what is known; scientists study what is not known. Scientists yearn for experimental results that contradict their established theories since such results are often the first step toward a new and better theory. Researcher Faye Flam states, "Ever more precise tests of the predicted particle masses and interactions have kept agreeing with theory, *to everyone's dismay*. 'At CERN [European Organization for Nuclear Research], they have been doing precision tests, *hoping that things wouldn't work*.'"[13] (emphasis added).

Why do contemporary homeopaths think that "science" means procedures and fixed rules? Homeopaths and many others in our society could well acquire this erroneous impression of science from their science classes in school.

PSYCHOLOGICAL FACTORS IN MISPERCEPTION

In addition to homeopaths' misunderstanding of science, some universal psychological factors contribute to the misperception that the remedies cause the cures.

Desire: Patients Want Homeopathy to Be Valid

For many patients, homeopathy is very appealing, so they want it to be valid. Why? The reasons can be grouped into three categories: (1) perceptions about homeopathy, (2) the physical process, and (3) the actual experience of the treatments.

Perceptions About Homeopathy:

- Homeopathy is a medical intervention that does nothing more than help our bodies heal themselves; it's natural, it's environmentally friendly, it's not high-tech.

- Homeopathy is perceived as risk-free, whereas conventional medicine is not.
- Homeopathy is gentle, unlike conventional medicine. There are few or no painful diagnostics or therapeutic treatments. There are fewer stressful and expensive hospital stays. Moreover, dissolving a sugar pill in one's mouth is pleasant and even easier than swallowing a regular pill. (Homeopathy is gentle in part because, appropriately, it often avoids treating conditions for which the only known effective treatments are not gentle by passing cases needing such care to appropriate specialists.)

The Process:

- The patient almost always gets some medicine, which is what most patients expect and want.
- The remedies are generally inexpensive, most can be purchased without a prescription, and the patients do not suspect that drug companies are making unreasonable profits.
- The process is active, not passive. The patient has control over his or her own care through the remedy-taking ritual, watching for changes, deciding when to take the next dose, and striving for a healthier lifestyle.

The Experience:

- The homeopathic practitioner is nonjudgmental, never denying or even questioning the patient's complaints and symptoms. The objective reality of the symptoms is usually irrelevant; homeopaths treat perceived symptoms. It is empowering to be heard and believed.
- The homeopathic practitioner is interested in *all* of the patient's concerns, not just the physical symptoms. The experience feels good to the patient.
- Some patients enjoy the counterculture aspect of "bucking" the dominant form of health care.
- The homeopath never dismisses a condition as psychological or psychosomatic, even if it is. Acceptance feels better than rejection or denial.
- Office visits are usually long, unrushed, and caring.
- Homeopaths attempt to explain fully how the remedy works and what to expect. This respect shown to the patient feels good, even if the patient does not fully understand the details.

• The remedies are individualized. Few patients take the same remedy even if they have the same primary physical symptoms. The patient feels special.

All this makes homeopathy so appealing that we want it to be valid. Unfortunately, such desire for validity usually clouds critical thinking. Facilitated communication, a technique that was supposed to help autistic children communicate, was enthusiastically practiced for a few years with almost no one asking whether it really worked. Later, testing showed that all the communications were in fact coming from the facilitators, not the children. Because everyone involved at the beginning deeply wanted to communicate with autistic children, few thought to challenge and test facilitated communication until sexual abuse allegations arose. Similarly, few homeopaths or patients want to challenge the validity of homeopathy.

The Habits of Mind of Professional Homeopaths

Homeopaths have instinctive feelings and reactions that tend to inhibit critical thinking. One of these feelings is missionary zeal. Homeopaths think, "The world needs us!" Homeopaths believe they have the best way to prevent human suffering, from traditional ailments and from new threats such as AIDS, radiation, potentially toxic chemicals in the environment, and terrorism.

Most homeopaths believe that homeopathy itself is a perfect system. When homeopaths feel insecure about a case or homeopathic theory, most will question (1) their own diligence, understanding, and training; (2) the patient's ability to communicate symptoms or to follow instructions; or (3) the accuracy and completeness of data in repertories and materia medicae. Homeopaths do not question homeopathy itself. This is understandable but fosters divergence of internal and external realities of homeopathy.

Homeopaths believe that more experience and study yields more success with patients; homeopathic masters are better than novices. In fact, the additional expertise may just deepen the misperception by providing more explanations for the failures and more techniques to try.

Homeopaths respect and admire members of their community who have charisma, eloquence, and confidence when they write, speak, and teach—those who create a strong inner reality in their readers, audiences, and students, not those whose work has external reality proven with hard data that demonstrate exceptional success in curing. Homeopaths value their internal reality over external reality, and they are not inclined to question and challenge their guru's claims of cured cases.

CONCLUSIONS AND THE FUTURE

Deceptions Are Common

If homeopaths have deceived themselves, they are not alone. It is natural for humans to be more influenced by personal testimonials, coincidence, rumor, emotion, and charismatic individuals than by solid evidence. The devotees of drinking radioactive water or breathing radioactive air (chapter 10) were passionate and sincere yet wrong about the health benefits of radioactivity. If the apparent power of homeopathic remedies turns out to be illusory, the longevity of the belief in the remedies stands out but has an explanation: homeopathy does indeed often improve people's health. The misperception is subtle, concerning only the cause of the health benefit, not the benefit itself.

Endorsements?

Some homeopaths feel that the increasing attention to homeopathy in medical schools is an endorsement.[14] A good physician should be informed about the other types of health care that patients may seek. The fact that medical schools may offer courses that include homeopathy does not prove that homeopathic remedies work. Similarly, having a CAM institute does not imply endorsement of CAM; it enables a medical school and its researchers to be part of the effort to determine which unproven alternatives are valid.

If HMOs and health insurers someday offer coverage for homeopathic treatment, this also will not necessarily be an endorsement of remedy activity for three reasons: 1. HMOs and insurers may recognize that because homeopathy as a whole helps many patients, they serve their customers and themselves by including homeopathy irrespective of the role of the remedies per se. 2. Because increasing numbers of their clients want homeopathy to be included, they may lose business if they do not include homeopathy. 3. They may include homeopathy because doing so saves them money (many fewer lab tests and relatively inexpensive remedies) as long as serious cases that may become much more expensive later are promptly referred to specialists.

Increasingly hospitals are offering CAM treatment. Beth Israel Medical Center has a full-time homeopath, not because the hospital believes homeopathy works, but because the hospital wants to offer what its customers want. It is a business decision; money talks. Dr. Matt Fink, former president and CEO of Beth Israel Hospital, frankly admits, "If hospitals don't get involved in these kinds of programs they will lose patients because patients will go elsewhere."[15] But there is a danger here that patients will assume that such hospitals believe all their treatments are effective. Do hospitals have an obligation to offer only proven treatments?

Future Research

Future research will clarify the status of homeopathy as a whole as well as the remedies themselves. There is considerable current research activity worldwide. In the U.S., the best chance for the needed funding is the National Institutes of Health's National Center for Complementary and Alternative Medicine (NCCAM), whose annual budget was $114 million in 2003. Clinical trials are so complex that those trained in research need to be in charge. Homeopathy is so complex that homeopaths need to be intimately involved in planning and participating in the research. Without this involvement, homeopaths can legitimately claim that some aspect of the homeopathic treatment in the trial was not properly done. The best procedure from all perspectives is to get agreement *in detail in advance* concerning all aspects of the tests. If the results on the role of the remedies is positive, the researchers and homeopaths will both be excited. If the results are negative, then researchers and healers can concentrate on homeopathy's other healing mechanisms to the benefit of all types of healthcare practice.

So What

If patients benefit, does it matter whether or not the improvement is due to the remedy itself? In some ways no. If a patient's health improves, the health-care method has value. Certainly, if patients use their own money, they have the right to select their own health care, but they should be reasonably well informed about the options and risks. However, when the cost is being shared communally through coverage by health insurance or HMOs, then economic and ethical issues become a more public concern.

Ethics

Would it be ethical to practice homeopathy if it were known that the remedies were not part of the cure? The practitioner could ethically say, "People who have been given this remedy in the past have usually felt better afterwards." However, the effectiveness of homeopathic care as a whole would suffer for two reasons: the placebo response would be weakened if the practitioner or patient doubted the remedies, and the homeopathic reason for lifestyle changes would not be as strong, since it would no longer be true that the remedy's action could be blocked by substances like coffee.

In practice, such problems are unlikely to arise. Belief is so strong that most practitioners and patients will continue to use homeopathy as they have always done even if the remedies are proven inactive to the satisfaction of the scientific world. Even if remedy bottles were required to display the warning, "There is no convincing evidence that this product is helpful," homeopathy would probably continue to thrive. "People are fed up with being passive recipients of authoritarian, paternalistic medicine," says alternative healer Dr. Andrew Weil. "And many of these [CAM] systems make people feel they are more autonomous, more in charge of their own destiny."[16] Even some people whose alternative treatments have failed continue to believe in the treatments because of the more attractive packaging and the real psychological benefits—they say they feel better, are happy, and feel confident their medical problem will be resolved. Many people clearly want more than a cure—they want a pleasant and caring experience. And perhaps above all else, they want hope. Physicians hesitate to offer hope where evidence of efficacy is lacking; CAM practitioners have fewer such inhibitions.

Importance of External Reality

Whether homeopathic remedies work is a question about external reality— it is a scientific issue and can only be settled by science. The evidence to date is not encouraging. Whether homeopaths want to continue to believe that their remedies are the cause of improved health is a personal issue. But when internal and external realities do not coincide, we may not achieve our objectives, whether they be building taller buildings or maximizing human health; the building may fall down, and our patients may not recover as quickly or permanently as might otherwise be the case.

Conclusions

Homeopathic theory is mired in two-centuries-old science and refuses to budge. Homeopaths cling to the concept of the vital force and miasms, ignoring the huge strides in understanding life and disease. Homeopathy has largely ignored the development of tools and techniques to establish cause in health interventions. It has been shown beyond all reasonable doubt that any approach other than random-assignment placebo-controlled double-blind clinical trials can easily deceive those involved. And yet the vast majority of homeopaths put their faith in cases, and as a result, they are probably deceived about the cause of patient improvement. Most of this inertia, this inability to utilize scientific advancements, can be attributed to homeopathy's reverence for its founder, Samuel Hahnemann. Homeopaths' blind faith in Hahnemann's teachings is like religious fundamentalism, with its acceptance of ancient written words as the highest truth.

The very foundation of homeopathy, the Law of Similars, which most homeopaths feel is a rock-solid, unquestioned law of nature, is in fact weak. It is so loaded with conditions, exceptions, and vague concepts that it is nearly unfalsifiable and hence nearly untestable. Homeopaths are convinced they see the law's verification daily through watching the progress of their patients. This is the primary source for their internal reality of remedy effectiveness. Homeopaths mistake plausible-sounding retrospective explanations of patient progress for scientific evidence of external reality. Scientific verification of a theory or law comes from making risky predictions—predictions that could be contradicted by facts. But the Law of Similars only predicts what might happen in individual cases, not what will happen. The retrospective explanations are more likely just an elaborate web of excuses to "explain" the lack of straight-forward improvement of many patients—excuses built up over time in a well-intentioned but self-deceiving attempt to save a health-care system that did not live up to its expectations, even though it unknowingly stumbled upon a number of features and rituals that in fact can assist healing.

POSTSCRIPT

If evidence generated after the writing of this book proves me wrong about the role of the remedies themselves, I will be delighted. When we scientists stick our necks out by making falsifiable and hence risky predictions, we enjoy the outcome no matter what happens. If we are right, we get a little ego boost. If we are wrong, we learn something we did not previously know or believe was true. Both experiences are positive.

NOTES

1. Wayne B. Jonas, "Alternative Medicine: Learning from the Past, Examining the Present, Advancing to the Future," *Journal of the American Medical Association* 280, no. 18 (1998): 1616–18.

2. Julian Winston and Chris Kurz, review of Rudolph Verspoor and Steven Decker's "Homeopathy Rediscovered: Beyond the Classical Paradigm," *Homeopathy Today* 20, no. 6 (2000): 17.

3. Noted American homeopath Constantine Hering (1800–1880) believed that farmers could rid their fields of weeds by spraying with a potentized remedy made from the weed seeds. Anthony Campbell, "Homeopathy in Perspective," chapter 7 [online], http://www.accampbell.uklinux.net/homeopathy/index.html [March 11, 2002].

4. Karl Sabbagh, "The Psychopathology of Fringe Medicine," *Skeptical Inquirer* 10, no. 2 (1985–86): 154–64; and E. J. Freireich, "Unproven Remedies: Lessons for Improving Techniques of Evaluating Therapeutic Efficacy," in *Cancer Chemotherapy: Fundamental Concepts and Recent Advances* (Chicago: Year Book Medical Publishers, 1975).

5. Some conventional medicines are similar, but in most cases there are falsifiable predictions concerning which outcome will mean success and which will mean failure. Also, many conventional medicines do not fit this dosing protocol; examples are antibiotics and preventive medications for heart attack patients.

6. Marcia Angell and Jerome Kassirer, "Alternative Medicine: The Risks of Untested and Unregulated Remedies," *New England Journal of Medicine* 339, no. 12 (1998): 839–41.

7. Stephen Barrett and William Jarvis, ed., *The Health Robbers: A Close Look at Quackery in America* (Amherst, N.Y.: Prometheus Books, 1993).

8. Julian Winston, "Why We Do It," editorial, *Homeopathy Today* 21, no. 9 (2001): 3.

9. Jörg Wichmann, letters to the editor, *Homoeopathic Links* 15, no. 3 (2002): 135.

10. Paraphrased from discussions during 2000 and 2002 on the Lyghtforce email list, archives online at http://www.lyghtforce.com/HomeoList.

11. Luc De Schepper, *Hahnemann Revisited* (Santa Fe: Full of Life Publishing, 2001), p. 26.

12. Maesimund Panos and Jane Heimlich, *Homeopathic Medicine at Home* (Los Angeles: J. P. Tarcher, 1980), p. 17.

13. Faye Flam, "The SSC: Radical Therapy for Physics," *Science* (1991): 254.

14. Bhaswati Bhattacharya, "Complementary and Alternative Medicine Courses Taught at U.S. Medical Schools" [online], http://www.rosenthal.hs.columbia.edu/MD_Courses.html [Nov. 15, 2002].

15. "The Alternative Fix" [online], http://www.pbs.org/wgbh/pages/frontline/shows/altmed/etc/synopsis.html [Nov. 2003].

16. Ibid.

Appendix 1:
Some Remedy Preparation Details

Remedy preparation is one of the few quantitative aspects of homeopathy. The overall guiding principle is that a 1X remedy involves using 1 gram (g) of the original material to make 10 milliliters (mL) of solution. If the starting material is adequately soluble, the procedure is self-explanatory.[1] The solvent can be alcohol (ethanol), distilled water, a mixture of the two, or glycerin. For plant remedies, the amount of plant material used is such that if it were dry,[2] 1 g would be used to yield 10 mL of solution. Similar guidelines are used for remedies made from animals or animal parts.

To prepare a solution from a gas, such as neon or hydrogen, some water or alcohol is placed in a bottle and the gas is bubbled through the liquid; succussion and dilution then follow. The general rule of using 1 g of original material to make up 10 mL of solution is inapplicable to gases; their solubility is too low.

If the starting material is an imponderable, such as x-rays or moonlight, a closed bottle of alcohol or water is exposed to the radiation; this liquid is then diluted and succussed. (The x-ray dose is 1000 Rad according to the HPUS.)

Preparation of decimal (X) and centesimal (C) remedies is described in chapter 1. Curiously, according to the HPUS, making centesimal remedies starts with making 1X and then 2X attenuations. This 2X attenuation is then called a 1C attenuation, and subsequent attenuations all involve dilutions of a factor of one hundred.

LM remedies are less common. They are diluted by a factor of 50,000 at each stage except the first. A 1LM remedy has been diluted by a factor of 250 million and has had one set of succussions. A 2LM remedy has been succussed twice and has a dilution of 50,000 times 250 million or 1.25 x 10^{13}. LM remedies are called *50 millesimal* remedies (or "Q remedies" in Europe). The specified dilution procedures for LM remedies involves wetting 500 pellets with one drop of the previous attenuation and dissolving one of those pellets in 2 mL of alcohol to make the subsequent attenuation, according to the HPUS.

Because of the three different potentization methods, and because of the range of potencies, a large number of remedies exists for each given starting material (see table A1.1).

Table A1.1. The Dilution of Remedies[a]

Number of Dilution Stages	X Remedies		C Remedies		LM Remedies	
	Designation	Dilution Factor	Designation	Dilution Factor	Designation	Dilution Factor
1	1X	10	1C	100	1LM	2.5×10^8
2	2X	100	2C	10,000	2LM	1.25×10^{13}
3	3X	1,000	3C	10^6	3LM	6.25×10^{17}
4	4X	10,000	4C	10^8	4LM	3.13×10^{22}
5	5X	100,000	5C	10^{10}	5LM	1.56×10^{27}
6	6X	10^6	6C	10^{12}	6LM	7.81×10^{31}
12	12X	10^{12}	12C	10^{24}	12LM	6.10×10^{64}
30	30X	10^{30}	30C	10^{60}	30LM	2.33×10^{149}
200	—	—	200C	10^{400}	—	—
1,000	—	—	1,000C (M)	$10^{2,000}$	—	—
10,000	—	—	10,000C (or 10M)	$10^{20,000}$	—	—
100,000	—	—	100,000C (or 100M, or CM)	$10^{200,000}$	—	—
1,000,000	—	—	MM	$10^{2,000,000}$	—	—

a. X and LM remedies are not commonly available in potencies over 30 and thus are not represented in this table.

In practice, some homeopathic remedy manufacturers have machines that do diluting and succussing automatically to make the higher potencies. Suppose that the machine has just finished succussing a 105C remedy. In one manufacturing method, the machine then removes the bottle seal and tips the bottle upside down. The contents go down the drain except for what sticks to the inside. The wet bottle is then turned upright, refilled with solvent, sealed, and succussed, resulting in a 106C remedy. The bottle size and procedural details have been selected so that the volume of remaining drops is $\frac{1}{100}$ of the bottle's full volume. This is the so-called **Korsakovian method**, the key being the reuse of the wet bottle at each stage. If new, clean, dry containers are used at each stage, the method is called **Hahnemannian**.

NOTES

1. If the solid's solubility is too low, 1 g is dissolved in enough solvent to yield 100 mL of solution, which is considered a 2X remedy.

2. If the original material is moist, its water content is taken into account so that the brew ends up with uniform alcohol content as well as the desired concentration of the original material.

Appendix 2:

Molecules Remaining in Dilute Remedies

F ew dilutions are needed before there are no original medicinal molecules left (see table A2.1). The usual statement is that remedies more dilute than 12C or 24X have little chance of delivering an original medicinal molecule in a dose, because Avogadro's number is 6×10^{23} or about 10^{24}, and a 24X remedy has been diluted by a factor of 10^{24}. This estimate is a simplification but conservative. Since the first step in remedy preparation involves a certain mass of the original medicinal material, the number of molecules will be larger if the mass of each molecule is smaller. The potency of remedies wherein the chance of retaining a molecule of the original material falls below 10 percent is illustrated in figure A2.1.

For example, the mass of one molecular unit of radium bromide is about 306 atomic mass units (**amu**). Using the graph, we find that one sugar pill of radium bromide remedy as dilute as 19X is unlikely (less than one chance in ten) to have any radium bromide left in it. The number of original molecules is greater in drops than in pellets because it takes much less than a drop (roughly $\frac{1}{40}$) to wet a #35 pellet when the pellets are medicated; thus for liquid radium bromide remedies, potencies of 20.7X and higher have less than a 10 percent chance of containing original molecules in a drop. (Although these potencies can be calculated with decimals, in practice such noninteger potencies are not made.) The molecular mass of sodium chloride (which homeopaths call Natrum muriaticum) is smaller, 58; thus there are more atoms for a given potency and higher potencies are needed before there is no sodium chloride present. Sodium chloride pellets or liquid remedies with potencies of 19.8X or 21.5X respectively have a 10 percent chance of containing one molecule.

Table A2.1. Number of Remaining Original Medicinal Molecules[a]				
Potency C	Potency X	Approximate number of original medicinal molecules per pill[b]	Number of pills needed for a reasonable chance of at least one original medicinal molecule	Volume of liquid remedy needed for a reasonable chance of at least one original medicinal molecule
1	2	10^{17}	1	<< One drop
6	12	10^7	1	<< One drop
12	24	10^{-5}	100,000	~2,300 drops
30	60	10^{-41}	10^{41} (nearly a billion times the mass of the Earth!)	10^{34} gallons (10 billion times the volume of the Earth)
100	200	10^{-181}	10^{181}	10^{174} gallons (much more than the mass of the known universe)
200	400	10^{-381}	10^{381}	10^{374} gallons "
1,000	2,000	$10^{-1,981}$	$10^{1,981}$	$10^{1,974}$ gallons "
10,000	20,000	$10^{-19,981}$	$10^{19,981}$	$10^{19,974}$ gallons "
100,000	200,000	$10^{-199,981}$	$10^{199,981}$	$10^{19,9974}$ gallons "

a. Because original concentrations of tinctures are not given in homeopathy—only the procedure for their preparation is specified—the numbers in this table are estimates, calculated for the particular case of a soluble compound with a molecular mass of 28 amu.

b. When the math says there are only a few molecules or less than one molecule left, the interpretation changes to a probability. For example, the math says that in a 12C remedy, there are $10^{-5} = 0.00001 = \frac{1}{100,000}$ molecules left, meaning that there is one chance in 100,000 of having a molecule.

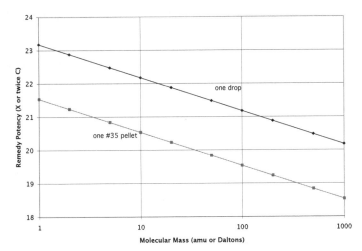

Figure A2.1. Remedy potencies for a 10 percent chance of a remaining original medicinal molecule. For potencies above the respective curves, there are essentially no molecules left in one pellet or one drop.

These examples and figure A2.1 assume remedies made of pure soluble materials; this condition yields the largest number of original molecules in remedies. For all other cases, the original material runs out sooner in the dilution process. Tinctures, like teas, contain only a small fraction of the original plant material. If 10 percent of the material were extracted, and if all the molecules had the same molecular mass, then the attenuation past which the probability of finding a molecule in a pill or a drop falls below 10 percent would be one X value less than in figure A2.1 since ten times less material is in the remedy.

For remedies made from insoluble solids such as gold and granite, the material, despite the grinding in trituration, does not dissolve but remains in chunks that are tiny by human standards but huge in terms of the number of atoms. Thus, it takes fewer dilutions before none is left. Suppose the particles of gold had 10^{12} atoms after trituration instead of single atoms as in solutions made from soluble materials. Then the critical potency is 12 X = values lower; therefore gold remedies would have no gold left (one chance in ten, or less) for potencies above 6X (or 3C) for a sugar pellet and above 8X (4C) for a drop of liquid remedy. For gases, the solubility in water is low,[1] so that a low initial concentration is unavoidable. Because some of the gas also escapes during exposure to the air during each attenuation, the original molecules will run out many attenuations earlier than in remedies made of soluble solids. For imponderables, no original material is left at any potency since there is no material to begin with.

For all LM remedies, original medicinal molecules are unlikely to be found in one pellet or one drop of 4LM or higher potency. For certain LM remedies, the original material may be gone at an earlier dilution stage.

NOTE

1. For the noble gases, mole fraction solubilities in room temperature water are on the order of 10^{-5} to 10^{-4}.

Appendix 3:
Water Clusters

As discussed in chapter 3, some researchers have hypothesized that remedies diluted beyond the molecular limit retain the healing information of the original medicinal molecules by virtue of water clusters, stable groups of water molecules that form structures around the original medicinal molecules and can exist and self-replicate in the absence of the original molecules. Homeopaths speculate that succussion helps them replicate, and their concentration is presumed to be higher in more potent (more dilute) remedies.

If memory is in water clusters, there must be at least millions of different cluster types given the potential for millions of different remedies postulated by homeopaths. Moreover, many single remedies will have thousands of distinct cluster structures because they consist of thousands of different compounds.

Many dilemmas arise in assessing the hypothesis of water clusters:

- If there is no limit to increases in potency, as some homeopaths claim, and yet the active ingredient is a water molecule cluster, we have a contradiction: An infinite number of water molecule clusters cannot be made from a finite number of water molecules. Perhaps homeopaths have not yet *observed* a potency limit.

- If the larger number of clusters makes remedies more potent, (1) then the size of the dose (e.g., how many pills) should make a difference, contrary to what many homeopaths claim, and (2) taking a larger quantity of a particular potency would be equivalent to taking a smaller quantity of a higher potency, again contrary to what homeopaths say.
- How do the water molecules know to make structures around the original starting material and not around the contaminants that enter at every stage of remedy preparation? (See appendix 4.) Or, how do our bodies know not to react to the clusters that represent the contaminants?
- How can clusters work for the imponderable remedies, which have no molecules around which clusters can form?
- In tautopathy, how do the clusters represent only the undesirable side effects but not the supposed healing aspects of the original material?
- How do clusters evaporate, as would seem to be required when the medication is taken by sniffing the remedy? Larger structures have much more difficulty evaporating.
- What would be the advantage of a single remedy containing 12C and 30C and 200C of the same remedy? If the active ingredient is clusters, then this combination would be equivalent to a single potency.
- Why would it be necessary to keep diluting past the molecular limit? Why not just succuss since succussion is claimed to create more clusters, whereas dilution wastes clusters? Ninety-nine percent of the clusters are poured down the drain at each dilution stage when C remedies are being made.
- If the water clusters hold the healing power, then how do remedies work that are not based on water, such as remedies in which the carrier is lactose, sucrose, alcohol, ointments, or rice paper? These media must carry the healing information even though they contain almost no water.
- Perhaps the water clusters do not evaporate from the wetted sugar pills—just the ordinary water or alcohol evaporates. If so, the mass of the pills must increase measurably for very high-potency remedies wherein many of the water molecules are locked up in the clusters. I predict that measurements will not confirm this mass increase.
- The process of trituration is believed to be as effective as dilution and succussion for potentizing remedies, but no water is involved at all. How can a water cluster theory explain the potency of triturated remedies or of remedies that use pure alcohol or glycerin as the solvent?

- Even just alcohol *vapor* must contain the healing information, according to some homeopaths, since actually wetting the pills is not necessary when medicating them; the vapor alone can do the job.[1] The active ingredient must be in the evaporated as well as liquid alcohol, yet when the alcohol leaves the pills as they dry before they are bottled, homeopaths believe it does not take away the active ingredient.
- Some homeopaths believe that provers who do not take the remedy get the same symptoms as those who do. Some homeopaths also believe that patients need not take the remedy to benefit from it. If so, it would seem that water clusters cannot be the correct theory. Or perhaps the clusters constantly radiate healing information.
- Some homeopaths claim that remedies become deactivated by certain storage conditions. Water molecule clusters might be expected to lose their structures at sufficiently high temperature, but why would they suffer from high humidity or from certain vapors outside the sealed remedy bottle?

In summary, the water cluster model seems to be contradicted by the claim of limitless potentizability, the existence of imponderable remedies, the claim that dilution is an important part of the potentization process, the claim that the number of pills taken at a time does not matter, the claim that remedies not based on water (for example, sugar pills) are supposed to work, the claim that for both provers and patients the remedy does not need to be taken to have an effect, the claim that certain storage conditions deactivate remedies, the claim that trituration increases potency, and the claim that sugar pills can be medicated by alcohol vapor alone. Many of these objections also apply to any theory based on matter. The overall conclusion is that either no material theory can be correct or that many fundamental tenets of homeopathy must be wrong. Homeopaths prefer the former and skeptics, the latter.

NOTE

1. Steven Kayne, *Homeopathic Pharmacy* (New York: Churchill Livingstone, 1997), p. 55.

Appendix 4:
Purity and Contamination

No substance or object that is *macroscopic* (large enough to be seen with the naked eye) is perfectly pure. One of the purest bulk materials prepared by humankind is silicon for electronics. Only about one atom out of every trillion is not silicon; however, a fist-sized piece of this purified silicon would contain roughly a trillion contaminating atoms. No manufacturing process can totally exclude impurities from entering the final product. Even triply distilled water is not pure; if it is or has been in contact with air, air becomes dissolved in it: if it is in a glass or stainless steel container, some of the glass or stainless steel dissolves in it. Modern laboratory techniques can show that nothing is perfectly pure.

How do nonhomeopathic manufacturers contend with this inevitable contamination? Whether they are making medicine or computer chips, they determine how much contamination of what kinds is tolerable (i.e., will not undermine the usefulness of their product), and design their procedures to meet the needed criteria. They can determine whether they have succeeded by directly measuring the contamination or measuring the effect on the functionality of the final product. For example, conventional medicines work as intended as long as there are enough medicinal molecules and sufficiently few interfering molecules.

Contaminants in homeopathic remedies come from three sources.

1. The raw medicinal materials used to make homeopathic remedies

cannot be perfectly pure. Flowers and leaves are "contaminated" with insect feces, dust, soot, volatile organic compounds, tars, viruses, fungi, bacteria, pollen from other species, comet dust, soil particles, decay products from radon, oils and dead cells from human skin, and fibers from fabrics. Washing can substantially decrease the amount of this contamination but cannot eliminate it. In fact, the washing itself adds contamination since truly pure water does not exist. There is always a little inevitable contamination.

2. The material and tools used during remedy preparation contribute foreign material. The water, alcohol, and lactose are not pure. Mortars and pestles are not perfectly clean; nor are the bottles, lids, and droppers, or pipettes used in the dilution process. In addition, even if all the manufacturing tools were perfectly clean, molecules from each of them will inevitably enter the remedy. All materials dissolve to some extent, and whenever any material is rubbed or even just touched, some of its molecules come loose. Thus porcelain, glass, and plastic molecules enter remedies during manufacturing.

3. All remedies are exposed to air during manufacturing, and all gases have some solubility in water. Thus all remedies contain all the gases in air (table A4.1) both in molecular and potentized form. In addition, air, no matter how carefully filtered, contains many more ingredients than indicated in table A4.1, some of which are contributed by human breath.

Table A4.1. Some of the Components of Clean Air[a]

Constituent	Content by Volume (percent)
N_2	78
O_2	21
H_2O	0.5–1
Ar	0.93
CO_2	0.037
Ne	0.0018
He	0.0005
CH_4	0.0002
Kr	0.0001
H_2	0.00005
N_2O	0.00005
Xe	0.000009

a. Values are approximate, and, except for water, are for dry air.

Does all this contamination matter? The answer is yes and no. Yes, it does matter from a molecular point of view, especially in the higher-potency remedies, because no original medicinal molecules are left; the contaminants dominate. But the alleged memory/energy of the contaminants is also strong. A 100C remedy will include dozens if not hundreds of different kinds of molecules that entered at each stage of attenuation, and memories of all of these at all potencies up to about 100C, plus memories of thousands more compounds at potencies of around 100C that entered with the original medicinal material. How does the remedy know to represent only the original intentional molecules?

Homeopaths would say that this contamination does not matter in practice. They claim that such inevitable contamination is taken into account in provings. Presumably the remedy used in the provings had the same contamination, and whatever effects it had were included in the provers' symptoms. This claim would make uniform manufacturing practices vital, and homeopathy puts much effort into achieving such uniformity.

Even if provings take this contamination into account, there is another problem. Remedies whose initial medicinal material is water or alcohol or some of the individual gases in air will be contaminated with each of the other materials. Thus, those remedies all should be closely related if not identical, with only a slight difference in potencies due to different concentrations of each material at the beginning of the process. Remedies nominally made from water, alcohol, oxygen, xenon, neon, and hydrogen should produce nearly identical symptoms, but homeopaths find them each to have a distinct set of symptoms.

Most of these problems arise because of homeopathy's belief that less is more—the most dilute remedies are the most potent. With such extraordinary dilutions, contamination and impurities are not only sometimes the dominant molecular ingredients (other than the carrier or base), but their theorized "water memory" or nonmaterial essence should also be nearly as strong as that of the intentional medicinal ingredients.

Two hundred years ago, Hahnemann and the world of science may not have understood the reality and pervasiveness of contamination, but now we do. Contamination matters in many industries, and these industries quantify and control it. Homeopathy seems ambivalent; it attempts to control contamination but rarely quantifies it, relying more on prescribed procedures than on measured results. Perhaps contemporary homeopaths ignore this kind of contamination because the situation is hopeless. There is no good reason why contamination shouldn't influence remedies, yet there is no way to eliminate all of it. Another homeopathic reason not to worry is that most patients improve, so the contamination problem cannot be important. Yet another reason might be that Hahnemann did not address it—he provided instructions for making remedies, so the method he described must be okay.

Appendix 5:
The Multitude of Procedures for Selecting the Remedy

I t is remarkable how many methods homeopaths use for selecting the remedy for a patient. In the summary presented in this appendix, the focus is on (1) the large number of methods rather than their details, and (2) the likelihood that different methods result in different prescribed remedies. The methods have been organized into two groups described in the two sections below.

CLASSICAL HOMEOPATHY: THE LAW OF SIMILARS AND THE TOTALITY OF SYMPTOMS

All classical homeopaths use the Law of Similars to select remedies. However, at every stage of the process, choices are based on philosophical preference and personal judgment. Perhaps this is why many homeopaths describe their profession as more of an art than a science, but the consequence is poor consistency among homeopaths.

Which Symptoms Happen to Be Mentioned During Interview

Different homeopaths ask different questions. Patients are not equally comfortable with different homeopaths. Interviews are not all the same length. The symptoms mentioned and the particular words used to describe them will vary, depending on the homeopath. Hence, different remedies may be prescribed. Conventional medicine has some of the same vulnerability, but its larger reliance on measurements and lab tests and the lesser value given to the patients' exact words or to mental and emotional symptoms results in more consistent prescribing.

Selection of a Subset of Symptoms

The patient interview may produce dozens to hundreds of symptoms. Homeopaths focus on a few, those believed to be the "characteristic," "strongest," "most clearly delineated," "essential," "dominant," most "vivid," most "complete" or those that best represent the "essence" or the "totality" or the "individual character" of the case or the "center of the case," or best express the disturbed equilibrium of the patient, or that are associated with a particular remedy and hence are "guiding" or "keynote." Since few of these terms are clearly defined, selecting symptoms is clearly subjective, increasing the likelihood of inconsistencies among different practitioners.

Vithoulkas further prioritizes the selected symptoms:

> The most characteristic symptoms are pulled out and arranged according to their importance. This must be done with extreme care, taking into account archical level, how strongly it represents the essential pathology of the patient, its timing in relation to the evolution of the current pathology, etc.[1]

Great care may be needed precisely because the criteria are so many and so vague; inconsistencies are inevitable despite the care.

Instead of selecting a small fraction of the symptoms, why not include all symptoms? What is gained by leaving symptoms out and then looking for the best remedy fit? Before the computer age, it was probably necessary to select a few symptoms just to make the task of finding the simillimum manageable. Perhaps that habit has now become ingrained, despite the advancement of technology.

Repertory Selection: Which Database?

There are many different repertories. Some are old classics or updated versions with "corrections" and edits. Others include very recent provings. Different translations of foreign language repertories are not identical. Some repertories have unusual organization. Each homeopath has favorite repertories. Some computer programs attempt to include every entry in every repertory; they also give the user the option of including or excluding proving data from particular sources. Clearly the selection of repertory will affect the final chosen remedy; if a repertory does not include a particular remedy or symptom or that remedy is not listed under an important symptom of the patient, it will not be selected; if a particular repertory uses different wording than the patient did to describe the symptoms, remedy selection can also be influenced.

Flat (or Neutral) Analysis

Once the most important symptoms and the repertory have been selected, the simplest strategy for finding the best remedy is to see which remedy is mentioned most frequently, in other words, which remedy has been observed to cause the largest number of the patient's symptoms. Homeopaths call such a choice a "flat" or "neutral" analysis. While the analysis may be neutral, the result is not since it is dependent on the case taking, the selection of the repertory, and especially on symptom selection.

Symptom Ranking

If a given symptom is especially strong for the patient, or if for any reason the homeopath believes it is more important, it can be given more weight. For instance, the homeopath can give each selected symptom a grade of 1, 2, or 3, with 3 corresponding to the strongest or most important symptoms. Then the practitioner (or the software) can quantify the remedies. Remedies associated with the more highly ranked symptoms receive a higher number. Each remedy's score is the sum of corresponding 1s, 2s, and 3s associated with the symptoms that the remedy covers, and the remedy with the highest score is considered the most likely to cure the patient. Another type of ranking involves picking a very small number of the most important symptoms and considering only those remedies that have all these symptoms for subsequent analysis.

Power to Induce or Cure Each Symptom

For a given symptom, the listed remedies need not be treated equally. Typically, repertories grade each remedy listed for a given symptom as low, medium, or high, depending on the strength of the association between the remedy and the symptom. Generally, if many provers had the same symptom, the ranking is higher, although some homeopaths prefer to use the intensity of the symptom rather than the number of provers with the symptom as their criterion. Also, if a few cases appear to have been cured using this remedy for this symptom, the remedy's grade may be elevated. Homeopaths do not agree on these rankings and may change them for their own purposes. However arrived at, these remedy gradings can be quantified and used to select possible remedies.

Large Versus Small Remedies

A large remedy (a *polycrest*) has a large number of symptoms. Such remedies often rank high; many of the patient's symptoms will be found to be associated with such remedies. Thus, polycrests are commonly prescribed.

Some homeopaths at times choose to exclude polycrest remedies from their selection process. Instructions for the software Cara say, "Sometimes you just have to get rid of that polycrest smokescreen in a case and get directly at those small remedies waiting to be used."[2] Why? There is no compelling reason for choosing small (few symptoms) rather than large remedies, but the fact that homeopaths may choose either is another reason different remedies may be selected for the same patient.

Multiple Simultaneous Approaches

In computerized systems, most of these many criteria can be applied simultaneously with different weightings selected by the user. Choosing the weightings suggested by a respected homeopath results in an "expert" approach. However, since different experts have different weightings, even expert approaches will not always agree with one another.

The Fitting

The job of selecting a remedy is still not complete. The last step is to consult the materia medica and read about each of the remedies that seem to be the best match. In this process, homeopaths sometime speak of checking that the "essence" of the remedy matches that of the patient. Perhaps the materia medica mentions symptoms that the homeopath thought minor and did not include in the repertorization, or includes symptoms that seem plausible for the patient. Although the process is a vague, intuitive, and unquantifiable, it is always the final step. According to Vithoulkas, "If the 'essence' of the remedy seems to fit the 'essence' of the patient, and if the bulk of the symptoms are covered, then the remedy can be given with confidence."[3]

Fitting is even more of an art for homeopaths that do not see cases as mere symptoms but as having "textures" and "flavors." Moskowitz states:

> As perceived through the totality of symptoms, the texture and flavor of illness form a complex and often tangled skein of psychological and physiological threads in which the former often provide the elements of continuity and meaning, either directly, as personal narrative, or more indirectly, as a bioenergetic core around which the psychosomatic details naturally group themselves.[4]

The fitting can result in the chief complaint not being part of the remedy picture. If a patient sees a homeopath for indigestion, the prescribed remedy need never have induced indigestion in a proving or cured it in any case. In this regard, Castro asserts:

> You have flu and are feeling restless, irritable, hot and bothered and extremely thirsty. You find that Sulphur comes up strongly for all your symptoms but isn't listed under Flu in the Repertory. The closest remedy is Bryonia but Bryonia isn't restless. Read through both remedy pictures to see which one fits best; it will probably be Sulphur—the one that does not have flu in its picture—in which case Sulphur will work more effectively because it covers the whole picture. If the strong general and emotional/mental symptoms point to one remedy, then give it even if it doesn't have your physical complaint listed in its picture.[5]

If the fitting process does not yield a clear result, the homeopath goes back to the beginning, perhaps starting with a different set of the patient's symptoms. He or she may even need to go back to the patient to check for additional symptoms.

OTHER REMEDY SELECTION METHODS AND ISSUES

Once we leave the castle walls of classical homeopathy, the surrounding fields are fertile with a cornucopia of remedy selection approaches and issues. And of course homeopaths disagree on the layout of the walls; many would have the walls enclose one or both of the first two approaches in this section.

Doctrine of Signatures

As discussed in chapter 2, the doctrine of signatures is a belief that there are cures in nature for all ailments and clues in nature as to what will work. The doctrine of signatures cannot yield reproducible results. Each remedy has many clues (e.g., color, shape, location, texture, pattern, hardness, function, internal parts, people's emotional reactions, history, and other associations) and each clue can be associated with many symptoms and ailments. Thus the process does not point to a unique remedy.

Etiology

Sometimes homeopaths choose to emphasize the perceived *cause* of the symptoms over the symptoms themselves. If a patient says, "I have had this symptom since . . . ," homeopaths will often infer that the stated event caused the symptom. Kent's repertory lists remedies under rubrics such as "ailments after anger," "ailments from excessive joy," "ailments after being embarrassed," and "ailments from disappointed love."[6]

A woman with hearing loss in her left ear and a "lump sensation" did not respond to a remedy based in part on these symptoms. Then the homeopath learned that these symptoms had started when she "suffered mortification at her ill treatment at the hands of the Italian police" after an auto accident. When the prescription was changed to reflect this event rather than her symptoms, she reportedly recovered.[7]

Homeopaths practicing isopathy also ignore the symptoms and prescribe a remedy made from the agent thought to have caused the disease. An example would be treating a patient whose skin is extremely sensitive to sunlight with Sol, a remedy made from sunlight.

Using tautopathy, a homeopath would select a remedy made from chemotherapy drugs to treat the side effects of chemotherapy; symptom matching is not used. Clearly, the choice to use etiology, as well as the particular variety of etiology, results in different remedies, not consistent prescriptions.

Remedy Families, Classes, Kingdoms, and Other Groupings

Remedies based on chemical compounds can be classified based on some of their chemical properties or the elements they contain. Remedies can be grouped according to their origins, such as plant, animal, mineral, and imponderable, or in more detail, as snake venom remedies or remedies from spreading and climbing plants. The possibilities are endless. Some homeopaths have reasons to specify or to exclude a remedy from a particular grouping, perhaps because the symptoms seemed snakelike (perhaps including snake dreams), or because of the patient's favorable or negative reactions in the past to a remedy from this group.

Some remedies are made from pure elements or from chemical compounds in which a particular element seems important. Homeopaths who think that chemical composition is significant may want to prescribe or exclude a remedy which contains a particular element. Other schools of thought lead homeopaths to focus on remedies related to a particular column or row in the periodic table.[8]

Themes

Sometimes homeopaths put extra emphasis on some common characteristic of the symptoms rather than the symptoms themselves. For instance, symptoms may be one-sided, all occurring on the left side of the body, in which case a remedy with very strongly left-sided symptoms might be chosen over another even if it does not cover the specific symptoms as well. Other themes revealed by the symptoms might be a tendency to excess (e.g., loquacity, perspiration, skin excrescences, heavy or prolonged menstruation), or to exhibit coldness (e.g., emotional coldness and cold extremities).[9] However, themes are not unique. Homeopathy can find many different themes in a case; data selection, interpretation, and the degree of abstractness of the theme are all variables.

There is a parallel ambiguity in determining the essences (or themes) of the remedies. Some homeopaths might believe that the essence of a remedy is pacifism, whereas others think it is anger, which are nearly opposites. Skeptics would interpret this contradiction as evidence that such essences are unreliable. However, some homeopaths are perfectly comfortable with such opposites and might say that the true essence of the remedy is concern about conflict, which encompasses both pacifism and in anger. A practitioner who goes down this path can almost always find a common theme covering both the patient and remedy, but the themes become broader, less specific, and hence more subjective.

Themes can seem to make sense in retrospect. However, it is questionable that a group of homeopaths would all come up with the same theme for the same patient or remedy and hence unlikely that they would prescribe the same remedy for a given case even if they all practiced theme prescribing.

Primary Physical Complaint

In clinical homeopathy, practitioners choose to prescribe based only on the main physical symptom of the patient. If the patient has a sore throat, the remedy will be one that has sore throats clearly in its symptom picture. Most over-the-counter remedies are also aimed at primary complaints. Clearly, prescribing on the chief complaint versus on the whole person usually results in different remedies.

Constitutional Prescribing

In *constitutional prescribing*, the remedy is matched to the normal, healthy characteristics of the patient. Those homeopaths who use constitutional prescribing will almost certainly come up with different remedies than those who do not. Even among those striving for the constitutional remedy, consistency is not assured since (1) constitutional type is such a vague concept, (2) constitutional types of individuals can change over time, and (3) the constitutional type can be masked by the illness. As Stephen Kayne puts it, "Phosphorus patients commonly take on the characteristics of a Sepia constitution when they are ill and depressed."[10]

The Central Delusion

Some homeopaths start with the symptoms that a classical homeopath might observe but do not use them directly to select the remedy. Instead they interpret the symptoms and use their interpretations to select a remedy. Divya Chhabra describes the technique:

> Dr. Sankaran was unfolding this idea, where the feeling, or state, became classified as a delusion: a false perception of reality. This false posture is like emotional baggage, it's an imprint on the mind and body, so that the person, no matter what situation in life, sees not that reality, but sees the situation within him. He reacts to those situations, from his own perspective, out of all proportion to the stimulus. If he has this inner delusion that he is in the jungle, and has fear of a lion, no matter what his situation, whether he has fear before an exam, or sees a cockroach on [the] floor, if there's a knock on [the] door, or even if he breaks up with his girlfriend, we must take the rubric: 'fear of lion', and 'sensation alone in the jungle'. If we take 'fear of exam' as central, we will miss the remedy, because we haven't understood the inner state or feeling. If his girlfriend

leaves, he has wide eyes of fear at being alone (in the jungle), not disappointment in love.[11]

If a patient is afraid of cockroaches, some homeopaths will use this symptom directly while others will use fear of being alone in the jungle instead, and still others will use something else entirely since there is so much latitude in selecting the central delusion.

Multiple Diseases, Layers, and Miasms

Patients can have more than one ailment at the same time. An example is a patient who simultaneously has arthritis and the flu, but in practice it is often unclear whether there is more than one disease. Homeopaths who decide that there are multiple diseases will sometimes prescribe for one disease at a time, that is, on a subset of all the symptoms. There are different ways to decide which disease to treat first. One choice might be based on the chronic versus the acute nature of the diseases. Some homeopaths believe that the diseases are layered and that the deeper layers cannot be reached or even perceived without first curing the outer layers. Ironically, homeopaths generally disdain the value of identifying diseases at all, whether single or multiple. They prescribe for the individual patient based on the total symptoms picture. The whole concept of layering could be viewed as another unprovable reason (excuse) for why patients do not always just get well.

In a sense, miasms (certain obstacles to cure) are a type of layering. If a homeopath is having difficulty finding the simillimum, "it may be impossible to cover the totality of the symptoms with one remedy. In such a case observe which miasm is, so to speak, on top and prescribe for the totality of symptoms of *that* miasm, and when these symptoms are cleared off, the layer beneath, representing, perhaps, another miasm, may be prescribed for."[12] The topic of miasms is very complex, and homeopaths do not always agree that a miasm is present, which miasm it is, or which remedy should be used to treat it. Some homeopaths do not even subscribe to miasm theory.

Unusual Remedy Selection Methods

As mentioned in chapter 2, some homeopaths use additional methods to select remedies, such as electrodiagnosis, dowsing, and kinesiology, for which there is no evidence of even self-consistency, much less consistency with more conventional methods.

Patient Compensation

Some homeopaths feel that the simillimum can be different from or even the opposite of the symptom picture presented by the patient if the patient is compensating for the true symptoms. R. Rose Nightingale states:

> One example of the compensated state is that of an Aurum metallicum patient who may not appear to be in the state brought about by the proving of Aurum metallicum, that of great depression, suicidal tendency and hopelessness. In fact, because the Aurum metallicum patient is compensating by overachieving and conscientious behavior, the classic proving picture would never be seen."[13]

Since homeopaths will not agree whether or not the patient is compensating, there is potential for different homeopaths to prescribe remedies with opposite symptoms for the same patient.

Acute Exacerbation of a Chronic Condition

Normally, a homeopath treats a patient with a chronic disease by taking into account the whole person. However, if some of the symptoms are more intense than normal, the homeopath may prescribe based primarily on these symptoms. This method will of course usually result in a different remedy.

Cross-Cultural Errors

Homeopathy is interested in *all* symptoms and puts much emphasis on non-physical, that is, mental and emotional, symptoms. With symptoms being so broadly and loosely defined, the distinction between symptoms and normal, healthy aspects of patients' lives becomes blurred. Thus normal aspects of people's lives may be misinterpreted as symptoms.

For instance, in some Asian cultures, if a woman were extraordinarily excitable and flamboyantly talkative, her behavior would be considered unusual and therefore conceivably a symptom of some disorder. However, if the patient were Italian, this behavior might be normal and would probably not be used to select a remedy. As another example, many Western homeopaths use strong body odor as a disease symptom; however, strong body odor can be normal in some cultures and hence not a disease symptom.[14] This can result in *cross-culture errors*. Even within a culture, a normal condition for an individual may be misinterpreted as a disease symptom if it is unusual in the culture as a whole.

Follow-Up Remedies and Remedy Relationships

James Tyler Kent said, "You may administer a dozen remedies without them [*sic*] having any effect."[15] Since "more often than not, a single remedy will not cure a case,"[16] most prescribing is for follow-up remedies. One approach is to assess the patient's current symptoms and determine a new simillimum on that basis, the same as for the first prescription. However, many other approaches unique to follow-up prescribing can be used.

Remedies are believed to have specific relationships to each other. A *complementary* remedy is one that will not disturb the action of the first remedy but will help it to finish its healing work. Some remedies *follow well*; thus, if the homeopath has difficulty in selecting the best remedy based on symptoms, then a remedy which is known as a good sequel for the initial prescription might be chosen. Some remedies are particularly effective in *series* triplets that must be given in one particular order, such as Calc. followed by Lyc. followed by Sulph.[17] An *intercurrent remedy* is said to restart a stalled case; thus if a particular remedy seems to cause only limited benefit, and repetitions of the same remedy still do not cure the case, then giving an intercurrent remedy (relative to the original remedy) may get the case going again so that returning to the original remedy may result in a cure. Intercurrent remedies are often nosodes. A *collateral* remedy "runs parallel to the remedy given previously."[18] An *antidotal* remedy is called for if the previous remedy has caused an undesirable effect. There are also *inimical* or incompatible remedies; if a remedy is followed by one that is inimical to it, the results are not good. Some remedy relations are both complementary and antidoting; when a remedy is followed by another, the other sometimes antidotes the first and sometimes helps the first.

All this complex detail may provide plausible-sounding retrospective explanations for how patients' illnesses evolve, but it contrasts starkly with the fact that clinical trials have yet to make a convincing case that any remedy has any effect. The cart is often in front of the horse in homeopathy.

CONCLUSION

Given the enormous variety of remedy selection methods, a group of homeopaths is guaranteed to select many different remedies for the same patient, even homeopaths practicing classical homeopathy. If all or even just half of these methods work (the selected remedy causes the patients to improve), the explanation within homeopathy would be extraordinarily complex. A more likely theory is that they all *seem* to work equally well because none of them do—the health improvements homeopaths witness are not caused by the remedies.

NOTES

1. George Vithoulkas, *The Science of Homeopathy* (New York: Grove Press, 1980), p. 210.

2. Instructions for Cara Professional (software), (Nottingham, U.K.: Miccant Ltd., 2000), p. 60.

3. Vithoulkas, p. 208.

4. Richard Moskowitz, *Resonance: The Homeopathic Point of View* (http://www.Xlibris.com, Xlibris Corporation, 2000), p. 32.

5. Miranda Castro, *The Complete Book of Homeopathy* (New York: St. Martin's Press, 1990), p. 23.

6. J. T. Kent, *Repertory of the Homeopathic Materia Medica*, enriched Indian ed., reprinted from 6th American ed. (New Delhi: B. Jain Publishers, 1998).

7. Sandra M. Chase, "Homeopathy for Serious Physical Pathology," *Homeopathy Today* 22, no. 1 (2002): 27.

8. Jan Scholten, *Homeopathy and the Elements* (Utrecht, Netherlands: Stichting Alonnissos, 1996).

9. Most of these examples are paraphrased from Jeremy Swayne, *Homeopathic Method* (London: Churchill Livingstone, 1998), pp. 100–101.

10. Steven Kayne, *Homeopathic Pharmacy* (New York: Churchill Livingstone, 1997), p. 106.

11. Divya Chhabra, quoted in Penny Edwards, "Finding the Innermost State through the Circle: Inspiration and Compelling Teaching from Divya Chhabra," *Homeopath* 84 (2002): 6.

12. Elizabeth Wright-Hubbard, *A Brief Study Course in Homeopathy* (St. Louis: Formur, 1997), p. 12.

13. R. Rose Nightingale, review of *The System of Homeopathy* by Rajan Sankaran, *Simillimum* 14, no. 3 (2001): 94.

14. Some of the examples in this section are adapted from Thom Namaya,

"Cross-Cultural Considerations in Homeopathic Practice," *Homeopathy Today* 21, no. 7 (2001): 34–35.

15. James Tyler Kent, quoted in David Sollars, *The Complete Idiot's Guide to Homeopathy* (Indianapolis: Alpha Books, 2002), p. 272.

16. Jay Yasgur, *Homeopathic Dictionary* (Greenville, Penn.: Van Hoy Publishers, 1998), p. 125.

17. Wright-Hubbard, p. 63.

18. Abdur Rehman, *Encyclopedia of Remedy Relationships in Homeopathy* (Heidelberg: Karl F. Haug Verlag, 1997), p. 19.

Appendix 6:
Clinical Trial Replications

For a few kinds of ailments, homeopathy has multiple clinical trials, including attempts at replication. Ultimately this is what is required to make a convincing case. Such sets of trials are discussed in this appendix. Some of the interpretations here are adapted from other authors, primarily Harald Walach and Wayne Jonas.[1]

Arnica is a remedy often prescribed for bruises, swelling, and bleeding. The meta-analysis conducted by Klaus Linde and his colleagues[2] included eight studies involving Arnica alone, and the patients receiving Arnica did worse than the placebo patients in three of the studies.[3] Two more recent reviews of Arnica studies did not demonstrate conclusively that Arnica was more effective than treatment with a placebo.[4] Thus, despite some positive trials, the research evidence for Arnica's effectiveness is not strong.

David Reilly and his colleagues conducted three trials on patients with allergic rhinitis (allergy-induced inflammation of the nasal mucus tissue).[5] Two of the studies concerned pollen allergies and used 30C remedies made from grass pollens; the third concerned mostly allergies due to house dust mites and used remedies made from this type of mite. The significant outcome was a subjective estimate of symptom severity. The results were positive for all three studies. Morag A. Taylor, David Reilly, and others conducted a subsequent study of patients with allergies to house dust, dust mites, feathers, or cats.[6] The test "was designed in response to a challenge from an independent clinical team to contest the evidence from the three preceding trials that homeopathic dilutions seem to differ from placebo." The authors concluded that the results "reinforce earlier evidence that homeopathic dilutions differ from placebo."[7] However, this test was not a repetition of the previous three:

- It concerned dust, mite, feather, and cat allergies, whereas the first two studies involved pollen.
- The improvement in subjectively perceived symptoms in the treated compared to the control group in the previous studies was not confirmed—the treated and placebo groups were indistinguishable using this outcome.
- Although a positive effect was seen in peak nasal flow, this parameter was not measured in any of the previous studies. The contradiction between the subjective symptoms and measured nasal peak flow casts some doubt on the value of the study's conclusions.
- There is some question concerning the usefulness of peak nasal flow:

  There is absolutely no information that this measurement means anything. In fact, peak nasal flows are simply too unreliable to be of any use as a clinical measurement. The nose is a dynamic structure that can change its characteristics within any given thirty-minute period. No one in clinical ENT [ear, nose, and throat] practice uses nasal peak flows anymore as a measurement of anything.[8]

- The authors stated that a greater number of participants in the homeopathically treated group than in the placebo group felt *worse* during the first half of the study, but they do not consider this fact to detract from the apparent effectiveness of homeopathy. In their view these worsenings were "aggravations . . . provoked . . . by homeopathy . . . and seemed to point to a good outcome"[9] because the patients subsequently felt better. Normally when patients in the treated group feel worse than those in the control group, the outcome of the study is considered negative.

Overall, this trial did not replicate the previous studies, nor was it convincingly positive.

No researchers unrelated to Reilly's group have replicated his trials and obtained the same positive results. George Lewith conducted a study of patients with allergy to house dust mites who received a 30C remedy made from dust mites.[10] Although the treated group did better than the control group, the treated group did not improve (the control group declined). This is certainly a mixed result, and in addition the study did not replicate Reilly's studies in many details. Studies in Norway using birch pollen remedies for birch pollen allergy sufferers also did not show a clear positive effect and were not a strict replication of Reilly's studies.[11] A more recent (2002) larger study by G. T. Lewith was negative: "Homeopathic immunotherapy is not effective in the treatment of patients with asthma."[12]

Thus, impressive as Reilly's four studies may seem to be, a possible interpretation is that the group has made some of the same mistakes four times. Only when these tests have been replicated a few times by independent researchers will the conclusions be reasonably convincing.

It should also be kept in mind that that none of these allergy studies has anything to do with classical homeopathy. They tested isopathy: The remedies were not individualized based on each patient's symptoms but rather were made from the presumed causative agent of the patient's symptoms. The only commonality with classical homeopathy is the use of potentized remedies, although this is an important commonality since the ability of nonmolecular remedies to affect health is a significant issue.

Using homeopathy for headache sufferers has at times seemed promising. In a study conducted by Brigo and Serpelloni, remedies were only partially individualized; they were selected from a small set of remedies with headaches as one of their symptoms.[13] This study produced such spectacular results that three independent efforts followed. T. E. Whitmarsh, D. M. Coleston-Shields, and T. J. Steiner closely replicated the original study but found no such spectacular effect; their results only hinted at statistical significance.[14] Harald Walach and others conducted a study with full individualization of the remedies and found no effect due to homeopathic remedies.[15] After the twelve-week double-blind study, eighteen patients continued in a year-long follow-up study[16] that was not blind. For this part of the trial, they knew that they were receiving real homeopathic remedies; thus the full potential benefit of classical homeopathy was available, including repeat visits, changed prescriptions, and a continuing placebo stimulus. Those not in this group of eighteen went about their normal lives. Some used homeopathy outside of the study, some used conventional therapies, and some sought no treatment at all. All patients filled out a six-week headache diary. Interestingly, those receiving no treatment did the best in terms of reported headache frequency, duration, and intensity. A Norwegian headache study found no improvement in the patients' perception of their health, but neurologists' ratings gave homeopathy a statistically significant result.[17] The inconsistency is not reassuring. Thus, the exciting first study has not been supported by the ensemble of subsequent studies, including one close replication, all conducted by researchers independent of the original group.

Similar problems have beset other studies. Promising initial studies either have been followed by inconclusive or negative studies or have yet to be replicated by independent researchers; an example of the latter are the childhood diarrhea studies by Jennifer Jacobs.[18] Thus, overall, there is no independently confirmed successful application of a particular homeopathic approach for any particular condition.

Most of these trials were designed only to test the effectiveness of homeopathic *remedies*, not homeopathy as a whole. By intent, any benefits from all the other healing mechanisms that are part of homeopathy were excluded. Thus the negative results do not necessarily contradict the positive impressions of homeopaths and patients in the real world.

NOTES

1. Harald Walach and Wayne B. Jones, "Homeopathy," in *Clinical Research in Complementary Therapies*, ed. George Lewith, Wayne B. Jonas, and Harald Walach (London: Churchill Livingstone, 2002), p. 237.

2. Klaus Linde et al., "Are the Clinical Effects of Homeopathy Placebo Effects? A Meta-Analysis of Placebo-Controlled Trials," *Lancet* 350 (1997): 834–43.

3. G. Ives, "Homeopathy Versus Orthodoxy: The Current State of Play," Blackie Memorial Lecture 1999, *British Homeopathic Journal* 89 (2000): 17–25.

4. Edzard Ernst, M. H. Pittler, "The Efficacy of Homeopathic Arnica: A Systematic Review of Placebo-Controlled Clinical Trials," *Archives of Surgery* 133 (1998): 1187–90; R. Lüdtke and J. Wilkens, "Klinische Wirksamkeitsstudien zu Arnica in homöopathischen Zubereitungen," in *Jahrbuch*, ed. H. Albrecht, M. Frühwald (Essen, Germany: Karl und Veronica Carstens-Stiftung, KVC Verlag Essen, 1999): 97–112.

5. David T. Reilly and Morag A. Taylor, "Potent Placebo or Potency? A Proposed Study Model with Initial Findings Using Homeopathically Prepared Pollens in Hay Fever," *British Homeopathic Journal* 74 (1985): 65–75; Reilly et al., "Is Homoeopathy a Placebo Response? Controlled Trial of Homoeopathic Potency, with Pollen in Hay Fever as Model," *Lancet* (1986): 881–86; and Reilly et al., "Is Evidence for Homeopathy Reproducible?" *Lancet* 344 (1994): 1601–1606.

6. Morag A. Taylor et al., "Randomized Controlled Trial of Homoeopathy

Versus Placebo in Perennial Allergic Rhinitis with Overview of Four Trial Series," *British Medical Journal* 321 (2000): 471–76.

7. Ibid.

8. J. Raso, "Homeopathy: 'If Less Is More, Is Nothing Best?'" *Priorities for Health* 12, no. 3 (2000): 35.

9. Taylor et al.

10. G. Lewith, "A Double-Blind, Randomized, Controlled Clinical Trial of Ultramolecular Potencies of House Dust mite in Asthmatic Patients," abstract, *Forschende Komplementarmedizin* 7 (2000): 46.

11. S. Aabel, "No Beneficial Effect of Isopathic Prophylactic Treatment for Birch Pollen Allergy During a Low-Pollen Season: A Double-Blind, Placebo-Controlled Clinical Trial of Homeopathic Betula 30C," *British Homeopathic Journal* 89 (2000): 169–73; S. Aabel et al., "Is Homeopathic Immunotherapy Effective? A Double-Blind, Placebo-Controlled Trial with the Isopathic Remedy Betula 30C for Patients with Birch Pollen Allergy, *British Homeopathic Journal* 89 (2000): 161–68.

12. G. T. Lewith et al., "Use of Ultramolecular Potencies of Allergen to Treat Asthmatic People Allergic to House Dust Mite: Double-Blind Randomised Controlled Clinical Trial," *British Medical Journal* 324 (2002): 520–23.

13. B. Brigo and G. Serpelloni, "Homoeopathic Treatment of Migraines: A Randomized Double-Blind Controlled Study of Sixty Cases (Homoeopathic Remedy Versus Placebo)," *Berlin Journal on Research in Homeopathy* 1 (1991): 98–106.

14. T. E. Whitmarsh, D. M. Coleston-Shields, and T. J. Steiner, "Double-Blind Randomized Placebo-Controlled Study of Homoeopathic Prophylaxis of Migraine," *Cephalalgia* 17 (1997): 600–604.

15. Harald Walach et al., "Classical Homoeopathic Treatment of Chronic Headaches: A Double-Blind, Randomized, Placebo-Controlled Study," *Cephalalgia* 17 (1997): 119–26.

16. Walach et al., "The Long-Term Effects of Homeopathic Treatment of Chronic Headaches: One Year Follow-Up and Single Case Time Series Analysis," *British Homeopathic Journal* 90 (2001): 63–72.

17. P. A. Straumsheim et al., "Homeopathic Treatment of Migraine: A Double-Blind, Placebo Controlled Trial of Sixty-Eight Patients," *British Homeopathic Journal* 89 (2000): 4–7.

18. Jennifer Jacobs et al., "Homoeopathic Treatment of Acute Childhood Diarrhea," *British Homeopathic Journal* 82 (1993): 883–86; Jacobs et al., "Treatment of Acute Childhood Diarrhea with Homeopathic Medicine: A Randomized Clinical Trial in Nicaragua," *Pediatrics* 93 (1994): 719–25; Jacobs et al., "Homeopathic Treatment of Acute Childhood Diarrhea: Results from a Clinical Trial in Nepal," *Journal of Alternative and Complementary Medicine* 2 (2000): 131–39.

Glossary

acute ailment: An injury or disease with a rapid onset and a short course, meaning the problem is self-limiting; it either spontaneously cures or the patient dies. The problem may or may not be severe as homeopaths use the term.

aggravation: A temporary worsening of the patient's condition in propitious response to the correct remedy.

allopathic medicine (conventional medicine): **Allopathy** is a word coined by Hahnemann to describe treatment of disease with remedies that do not produce the disease symptoms in healthy people, in contrast to homeopathic remedies. The term is still used today, primarily in a pejorative sense by advocates of complementary and alternative medicine (CAM) to describe conventional medicine.

amu: Atomic mass unit, defined to be one-twelfth the mass of a C-12 atom. The most common type of hydrogen atom has a mass of approximately 1 amu.

antidoting: (1) Inhibiting the beneficial effects of a remedy by patient actions such as ingestion of certain foods or beverages, exposure to certain fumes, or exposure to certain other health care interventions. (2) Reversing unwanted effects of a remedy by treating the patient with another remedy or by the ingestion of certain foods or beverages by the patient.

applied kinesiology: The use of muscle strength testing to determine the medicinal or nutritional needs of patients. The patient might hold a candidate remedy in one hand while the strength of the other hand or arm is tested; if the patient's body needs the remedy, the patient's muscles allegedly show more strength.

attenuation: (1) The process of dilution plus succussion (or trituration) used to create the next higher potency of a homeopathic remedy. Synonymous with *potentization* and *dynamization*. (2) The product that results from each attenuation.

C: Roman numeral for 100, part of the designation of *centesimal remedy* potency, as in 30C.

CAM: Complementary and alternative medicine.

case taking: The gathering of all the patient's symptoms, primarily through interviewing the patient.

case: (1) The patient. (2) The facts about a patient that are needed for prescribing. (3) An account of a patient's symptoms, the treatment, and the outcome.

centesimal remedies: Remedies prepared with a factor of 100 liquid dilution at each stage of attenuation.

characteristic symptoms: Symptoms that tend to be unique to the patient and the patient's expression of the disease and hence tend to individualize the case and point to a single remedy. (See *strange, rare, and peculiar symptoms*.)

chief complaint: The symptom/injury/illness that was the primary reason for the patient to seek professional homeopathic help.

chronic condition: A disease or other ailment that is long lasting or recurrent.

classical homeopathy: Homeopathy as described by the old masters, principally Samuel Hahnemann. The single most important aspect is the *Law of Similars*. Other aspects often included are the *minimum dose*, the *single remedy*, and *individualization*.

clathrate: (See *water cluster.*)

clinical homeopathy: Single homeopathic remedies prescribed based on diagnosed illnesses or single symptoms, as in conventional medicine.

clinical significance: A concept related to the size of the health benefit of an intervention.

combination homeopathy: The use of standard mixtures of remedies to treat a single symptom or group of related symptoms.

common symptoms: Symptoms that are normally associated with a particular illness and hence tend not to be useful for individualizing the case.

complex homeopathy: Synonymous with *combination homeopathy.*

concomitants: Symptoms that occur in conjunction with the chief complaint.

constitution: The "symptoms" and general characteristics of a healthy person, including personality and physical appearance. People's constitutions are thought to correspond to particular homeopathic remedies.

constitutional remedy: A remedy matching a person's constitution. Such remedies are thought to improve the person's general well-being, increase resistance to disease, and help recovery from disease.

conventional medicine: The science-based health-care practice prevalent in the Western world; sometimes called "Western medicine." Use of the term *Western medicine* is inappropriate in this book because homeopathy is also Western.

crude dose: A dose of the original starting material itself, as opposed to its potentized forms.

cure: As used in this book, a significant improvement in a patient's physical and/or mental condition. Homeopaths distinguish between a true cure and an apparent or temporary or partial improvement; this book does not.

decimal remedies: Remedies prepared with a factor-of-ten dilution at each stage of attenuation.

doctrine of signatures: The theory that nature provides cures for most ailments, and gives clues to identify what should cure what. The clues are usually related to appearance or function.

dowsing: In homeopathy, the use of a small, handheld pendulum to help determine the appropriate remedy and/or potency for a patient based on the motion of the pendulum.

dynamization: Synonymous with *attenuation* and *potentization*.

electrodiagnostics: Use of electronic devices to help determine the appropriate remedy.

epidemic hysteria: The phenomenon of a number of people, often in the same geographic area, such as at a school, having similar symptoms wherein the cause is psychosomatic.

external reality: The physical world as known through the methods of science, as opposed to the world as perceived and felt by individual people.

false memory: A memory of an event that did not occur. The memory feels real to the holder and presumably is biochemically indistinguishable from ordinary memories. It can be created by a dream or by psychological conditioning.

false positive: In this book, an apparent but untrue cause-and-effect relationship, such as a statistically significant positive result in a clinical trial that was due to chance alone, or proving symptoms incorrectly attributed to the remedy.

fluxion method: A remedy preparation method involving continuous-flow dilution until the final dilution stage is reached, when the solution is succussed.

g: Abbreviation for *gram*, a unit of weight measurement. One ounce is about 28 grams; one pound is about 454 grams.

general symptoms: Symptoms that are not localized in the body, such as fatigue, anxiety, or euphoria.

grafting: Expanding the supply of a remedy by mixing as little as a single pellet with hundreds or thousands of unmedicated pellets or plain sugar; each pellet or grain of sugar is then thought to be as potent as the original remedy.

Hahnemannian method: A method of preparing *centesimal remedies* using a new bottle at each attenuation stage. Since making a 20,000C remedy would require 20,000 bottles, this technique is rarely used for higher-potency remedies.

healing crisis: A worsening of symptoms or the appearance of new symptoms in accordance with an aggravation, or *Hering's Laws*, as a desirable part of healing.

Hering's Laws: The types of patient responses to a remedy that indicate to a homeopath that the remedy is having a beneficial effect. These favorable responses involve the symptoms moving from inside to outside the body, moving down the body, moving from more to less important parts of the body, and revisiting old symptoms in reverse order of their original occurrence.

HMO: Abbreviation for health maintenance organization.

homeopath: A person who practices homeopathy. The formal education of people who call themselves homeopaths ranges from very little to Ph.D.s and M.D.s. Some have formal education in homeopathy and some have none. There are no generally accepted training, degree, or certification requirements for homeopaths. Thus the term *homeopath* as commonly used is only loosely defined. Some homeopaths would like to restrict the term to those who practice classical homeopathy.

homeopathic immunology: The prevention of future diseases by administering a homeopathic remedy derived from the disease or symptomatically related the disease. Also called *homeopathic prophylaxis*.

homeopathic pathogenic trials: A more contemporary term for *provings*.

homeopathy: An approach to health care based primarily on the *Law of Similars*, the concept that a patient can be cured with properly prepared minute doses of a substance which, when given to healthy people, induces the patient's symptoms. Homeopathy is not herbal medicine or acupuncture or any other CAM except homeopathy.

hormesis: the effect of a toxic material in high doses being protective or otherwise helpful in low doses.

HPUS: The *Homeopathic Pharmacopoeia of the United States*, the official U.S. certifier of homeopathic remedies and manufacturing practices.

imponderable remedy: A remedy whose starting material is not constructed of atoms or molecules. Examples are remedies made with light and magnetism.

inadvertent proving: An unintentional proving; a patient's getting additional symptoms characteristic of a remedy in a situation in which relief from symptoms was the intention.

individualization: Selecting the remedy and its dosing based on all the symptoms of the individual patient, as opposed to treating an identified disease or condition. As a consequence, patients with the same disease (as identified in *conventional medicine*) usually do not receive the same homeopathic remedy.

internal pharmacy: Natural biochemical mechanisms within human bodies that make chemical agents in response to people's mental states; agents that affect health positively or negatively.

internal reality: An individual person's perception of the world. (See *external reality*.)

isopathy: Treating patients with homeopathic remedies made from the agent that caused the illness.

Korsakovian method: A method of preparing *centesimal remedies* using a single bottle for a series of attenuations. The bottle size and procedure allow $\frac{1}{100}$ of the contents to remain when the bottle is emptied, so that when the bottle is subsequently refilled with solvent and succussed, the next higher attenuation is achieved.

large remedy: A remedy with a large number of symptoms. Synonymous with *polycrest*.

Law of Similars: The central homeopathic principle of "like cures like;" a remedy which can induce symptoms in a healthy person and can cure those symptoms in a sick person.

layers of disease: A homeopathic theory that diseases can be layered in the sense that the outermost layer must be cured first to reveal and treat the next layer.

LM: A designation for remedies prepared by a different technique than are X or C remedies and involving dilution by a factor of 50,000 at all but the first stage of attenuation.

M: Roman numeral for 1,000, used by homeopaths for a shorthand designation of *centesimal remedies* of 1,000C and beyond, e.g., 100M designates 100,000C and 20M designates 20,000C. MM designates 1,000,000C.

materia medica: A compendium of remedies and their associated symptoms.

memory of water or **water memory**: The theory that since no original medicinal molecules are left in many homeopathic remedies, the water of the remedy must have memory of the original molecules, and this memory can bring about cures.

meta-analysis: A statistical technique of pooling data from separate studies, such as clinical trials, and attempting to come to an overall conclusion based on the combined data.

miasms: Certain blocks to health, obstacles to cure, or predispositions to disease that are due to heredity, medical history, or environment.

minimum dose: The concept that the "smallest amount" of effective medicine is best.

mL: Abbreviation for *milliliter*, a unit of liquid measurement. One teaspoon is about 5 mL, and one cup is about 237 mL.

modalities: The conditions that exacerbate or ameliorate a particular symptom or group of symptoms, such as weather, exercise, body position, or food.

molecular dose: A homeopathically prepared remedy which has sufficiently low dilution that there is a reasonable chance of getting some of the original medicinal molecules in a dose.

mother tincture: (See *tincture*.)

multiple outcomes: More than one outcome in clinical trials. A trial with two outcomes might assess the patients' temperature and blood pressure twenty four hours after the treatment. A trial with four outcomes might assess the patients' temperature and blood pressure twenty four and forty eight hours after the treatment.

nocebo response: Ill health resulting from the expectation of ill health.

nonmolecular remedy: A homeopathically prepared remedy which is so dilute that there is little chance of getting any of the original medicinal molecules in a dose. Also called *ultramolecular.*

nosode: A homeopathic remedy prepared from diseased material.

original medicinal molecules: Molecules of the material used to make the remedy and after which the remedy is sometimes named, such as the molecules from the Belladonna or Arnica.

palliation: A reduction in pain and suffering without the cause being removed. Palliation is considered desirable if a cure is impossible; otherwise it is considered undesirable and is called *suppression.*

placebo: (1) An object or event in a healing environment that enhances the patient's belief that a health treatment will be effective. (2) A look-alike but inactive treatment (e.g., blank pill) used on the control group in clinical trials or given to patients who expect medicine but do not need any medicine.

placebo response: A positive effect on physical and/or mental health in response to the patient's expectations.

plussing: Expanding one's supply of a remedy or increasing its effectiveness by adding a small amount of it to a quantity of water. If the water is then stirred or shaken, the result is thought to be more potent than the original remedy.

polycrest: A remedy with a relatively large number of symptoms and hence homeopathically suitable for a wide range of ailments.

potency: The "strength" of a homeopathic remedy, based on the number and type of dilutions-plus-succussions (or triturations) used in its preparation. In homeopathy, the most dilute remedies are the most potent.

potentization: The process of successive dilutions and succussions (or *triturations*) used to make homeopathic remedies. Synonymous with *attenuation* (definition 1) and *dynamization*.

primary and secondary symptoms: Symptoms and their opposites in provers caused by the same remedy, such as constipation and diarrhea.

provers: People who participate as subjects in a *proving*.

provings: The process of giving homeopathic remedies to healthy volunteers and recording and analyzing their symptoms in order to determine what symptoms the remedy is capable of curing.

p-value: A statistical concept; a p-value of 0.05 or less is a common definition of *statistical significance* and means that there is a 5 percent or less probability that the results were due to chance alone.

radionics: A method of making homeopathic remedies involving placing a bottle of water or unmedicated pellets on a card with a complex pattern drawn on it.

random assignment: In clinical trials, a procedure to determine which volunteers are put into which group (treated or placebo) that assures randomness in the selections.

RCT: Abbreviation for *randomized controlled trial*, which is shortened from *random-assignment placebo-controlled clinical trial*. RCTs are considered by scientists to be the best way to determine the effects of medications and other interventions.

regression to the mean: In the context of health, the statistical tendency for symptoms to wane after they wax (and wax after they wane), assuming some random variation in symptom intensity.

remedy picture: The set of symptoms a remedy is thought to produce in healthy people, as gleaned primarily from provings.

repertory: An organized listing of symptoms with the remedies that produce them. A repertory contains essentially the same information as a materia medica but is organized by symptom rather by remedy.

rubric: A symptom as listed in a *repertory*. The symptom is crafted or word-smithed to fit the organizational scheme of the repertory.

sensitivity: The proclivity of people to react to homeopathic remedies. Some people are thought to react more strongly overall to a remedy; others are thought to have symptom-specific reactions.

simillimum: The remedy whose symptom picture most closely matches that of the patient and hence is most likely to bring about a cure.

single remedy: The homeopathic concept that only one remedy should be given at a time. The patient's reaction should then be observed over some time before deciding if a different remedy is appropriate.

small remedy: A remedy with relatively few symptoms, in contrast to a *polycrest*.

spaghetti effect: A term coined by the author to indicate a patient's getting well as the result of a physical or chemical factor not yet known to science. This unrecognized factor might be an herb in spaghetti sauce, a type of exercise, an environmental factor, or a side effect of another treatment.

statistical significance: A concept related to the reliability of conclusions, related to the probability that an outcome could be due to chance alone. In a clinical trial, if the number of people getting better after treatment has less than one chance in twenty of occurring by chance alone, often it is considered *statistically significant*, suggesting but not proving that the improvement was caused by the treatment.

strange, rare, and peculiar symptoms: Patient symptoms that are so unusual that they may be associated with only one remedy and hence may point to a *single remedy* as the *simillimum*. Strange, rare, and peculiar symptoms are "characteristic" symptoms.

succussion: The shaking of a diluted homeopathic solution, usually in a particular manner, believed to be important for making the remedy more potent.

suppression: The temporary lessening or transformation of symptoms in opposition to *Hering's Laws*, allegedly caused by an inappropriate remedy or dosing. Suppression is not considered desirable. (See *palliation*.)

symptom: In homeopathy, symptoms are defined very broadly. In addition to conventional physical symptoms, homeopaths include general, emotional, and mental symptoms, and include as symptoms what many people would consider to be normal traits. Examples of homeopathic symptoms include sore throat, desire for sweets, difficulty sleeping, and claustrophobia.

symptom picture: The set of symptoms for a particular patient.

tautopathy: Treating a patient who is taking a conventional drug with a homeopathically prepared remedy made from the conventional drug in order to alleviate the drug's side effects.

tincture: A relatively concentrated water/alcohol extract of a plant or animal (whole or parts) that is an early stage in preparing typical homeopathic remedies.

trituration: A method of preparing homeopathic remedies involving grinding and mixing with lactose.

vital force: The spirit or energy that homeopaths claim animates the physical body.

water clusters: Alleged self-replicating water-molecule structures that are stable up to at least 100° Fahrenheit, which are different for each homeopathic remedy, and which stimulate human bodies to cure themselves. Also called *clathrates*.

water memory: (See *memory of water*.)

whole person: Every aspect of the patient—physical, mental, and emotional. Because homeopathy treats the whole person, remedies are *individualized*.

X: Roman numeral for 10, part of the designation for decimal remedy potency, as in 6X.

Index

Page numbers for definitions are in boldface.